RECLAIMING
FEMININE WISDOM
AN EMPOWERING JOURNEY WITH ENDOMETRIOSIS

MELANIE ROSSITER

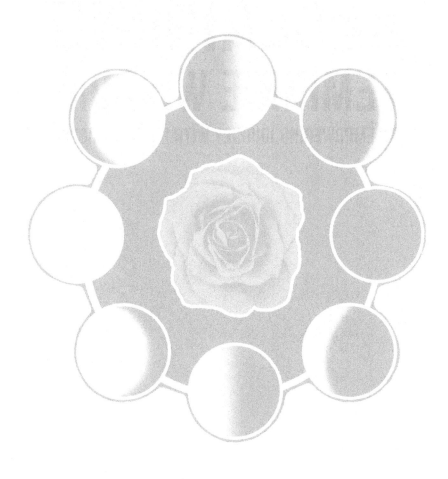

TABLE OF CONTENTS

CAUTION/DISCLAIMER

PLEASE MAKE SURE that you always obtain professional medical advice by consulting a medical practitioner. The information in this book should not be used as a substitute for professional advice. Any conditions requiring diagnosis or involving symptoms need review by a medical physician or doctor. Carrying out any of the practices or use of information in this book is at the reader's risk and discretion. The author or publisher cannot be held accountable for loss, damage or claims arising from use or misuse of suggestions set out in this book. Neither the author nor the publisher can accept legal responsibility or liability for any errors or omissions made that were believed to be true at the time of publication. Any practitioners mentioned in this book are done so in good faith. If you follow up with these practitioners, it is at your own discretion. When I use the words 'heal' or 'healing', I am not talking about curing something. I truly benefited from all these practices beyond what I could have hoped for and I know how transformative this work is for women, both for myself and in my work. Sending you love for where you are currently at.

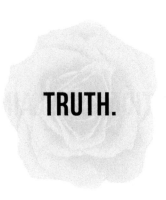

TRUTH.

"I think midlife is when the universe gently places her hands upon your shoulders, pulls you close, and whispers in your ear: I'm not screwing around. It's time. All of this pretending and performing—these coping mechanisms that you've developed to protect yourself from feeling inadequate and getting hurt—has to go. Your armour is preventing you from growing into your gifts. I understand that you needed these protections when you were small. I understand that you believed your armour could help you secure all the things you needed to feel worthy of love and belonging, but you're still searching, and you're more lost than ever. Time is growing short. There are unexplored adventures ahead of you. You can't live the rest of your life worried about what other people think. You were born worthy of love and belonging. Courage and daring are coursing through you. You were made to live and love with your whole heart. It's time to show up and be seen."

—Brené Brown,
Research Professor, University of Houston

This quote from Brené Brown, who studies courage, vulnerability, shame, and empathy, appeared as I was writing this book and feeling vulnerable about sharing my story. It's a long quote to use for the beginning of a book, I know, but I have received this wisdom on my own journey to a place of empowerment with endometriosis. I have learned about being true to yourself and the importance of sharing our authentic voice in order to heal and to be witnessed, heard and seen. The true strength is in acknowledging and sharing our vulnerability. It is through this that we can truly connect to one another and help to abolish unwarranted shame. So often, we hide parts of what make us human in a society that views feelings like vulnerability as a weakness and teaches us that it's best to stay silent through a misguided sense of protection. This hides our voices and disconnects us from our wisdom, truth and commonly shared experiences. Too often I see women in my work who are victims of trauma that they've felt unable to share and so have turned it inwards, making them feel trapped. Any sexual, cultural or emotional abuse they begin to feel had something to do with them, hence a manifestation of incorrect thinking and shame. It is shame that I feel can potentially block access to our emotions; we are conditioned to an extent that being seen as emotional and vulnerable is largely unaccepted or flawed. My journey highlighted how damaging this can be.

We need to break down the boundaries and walls we have built to protect ourselves from feeling emotional pain or rejection, without worrying about being judged or criticized. We often just want to be truly heard. The truth is that we only hurt ourselves when we deny our authenticity and our voice. But when we do connect to our truths and share them, we pave the way for others to do the same. So, here is my truth.

This book will support all women (particularly those of you with endometriosis or other menstrual conditions) through discussing feminine healing practices, spirituality, nutrition, and other holistic routes to wellness, and will help you to connect to your body's own inherent wisdom. Particularly with regard to menstrual cycle awareness and your cyclical rhythms and inner process.

You can use the book as a guide, dipping into chapters that are relevant at various stages of your life. However, I would recommend reading this from start to finish first as you will see how my journey unfolded, and how my story is interwoven throughout.

I began tapping into the power and healing wisdom inherent in the menstrual cycle; and a series of synchronicities led me to the right teachers, therapies, and books when I needed them. You often hear when the student is ready, the teacher appears. I began a quest that led me on an empowering healing path, delving into the feminine mysteries and questioning the effects of a historical patriarchal system on us all. In particular regarding women's healthcare, since I had what is likely one of the most common diseases that so few have heard of.

I will be including the methods I used and the experiences I had whilst discovering the gifts of my menstrual cycle and reconciling the lost respect for the feminine within myself.

WHERE IT ALL BEGAN.

MY STRUGGLE BACK to health began two weeks after the birth of my second child. I had to have postnatal emergency surgery for a retained placenta, which was followed by pain, adhesions (scar tissue sticking tissues or organs together), and endometriosis.

All this happened whilst attempting simultaneously to look after my new-born and one year old. At the time I kept a big smile on my face, replying, "everything's fine" to the outside world, whilst my health began disintegrating before me. Not to mention the cascade of hormonal fluctuation from having two children so close together, I wondered if I was literally losing my mind; I would find myself half way through a sentence and completely forget what I was going to say.

There was no time to process the trauma from my postnatal experience, and so it just dripped out over the coming year, with unexpected twists and turns, and eventually some amazing gifts arose from the experience.

Prior to having my children, I had always had some degree of pain around my periods, but I managed them fine, and they never altered my life. It was only before the birth of my first child that they were becoming increasingly more painful. I was very lucky to conceive both of my boys quickly as it was beginning to look like I had endometriosis. Whilst pregnant, there was no pain because my periods had ceased, although this isn't always the case when pregnant for all with the condition.

My mum had also had painful periods, and I was led to believe it was normal and told to take painkillers as that was what my mum did when she had her period. This is a story that plays out in many households around the world. My grandma had painful periods and so menstrual health was an issue that played out with the women in my immediate family, and I'm not sure how far back through our ancestral line. Women have painful periods, right?

Well no, pain whilst menstruating is not normal, this was a revelation for me. Throughout my teenage years and twenties, there was usually a degree of discomfort or pain, depending on the month, but luckily, at this time it didn't have any control over how I lived my life.

If you grow up believing that periods are supposed to be painful and this is true for you in your experience, you do not question it. I had no education on what having painful periods meant from a holistic or medical point of view, I just thought it was what happened to all women.

The wake-up call post-birth of my second child happened after continually going into triage in hospital with jelly-like pieces of tissue from my womb; I did not realise that this was placenta at the time. I wasn't sure because I had been told after birth that my placenta had all come out, the midwife even offered to show it all to me after the birth. We were always told to go to triage if we had any postnatal bleeding or problems, but I was repeatedly told to go home and wait to see if it would clear on its own. Eventually I ended up feeling I needed to push for a scan as my intuition was telling me something serious was going on and the wait-and-see approach was beginning to wear thin.

Finally, after a few visits, one of the doctors agreed I needed a scan and he began to take it more seriously. He said he would put me through as an inpatient rather than an outpatient to try and speed up the process. The doctor was pushing the radiology department for it urgently but they kept replying that they were very busy; but I was on the list. He told me it was likely to be around five days before I would be seen.

I am still shocked looking back at this. I should have taken myself into A and E. However, because I did not at this point class myself as an emergency, I didn't go. I did not want to waste their time if I was wrong, and at that time I didn't feel that I was in an emergency situation to the point where it could be life threatening. To be fair to the doctor, he did say I could try going to A and E, but it was more of a suggestion than something I needed to do.

I did not realise the risk I was taking by waiting, and lo and behold on day four I went into hospital with another section of placenta and was incredibly "lucky" that I was in hospital because when I went to the toilet, I began haemorrhaging and, before I knew it, I was shaking on a trolley with doctors pushing needles into my arm and an emergency operation ensued. It's amazing what you remember when you go into shock, I remember the dingy hospital lights blaring at me and the doctors voice which seemed to fade into the background of the commotion.

He told me "everything will be fine, you are in the right place" and I remember picturing my newly born son and thinking that I didn't have time for this, I needed and desperately wanted to be with him. I couldn't understand why it was happening and I felt frustrated that I'd made it clear that there was a problem before, why had no one really listened?

The significance of my body waiting for the exact moment I could get help quickly was not lost on me; I was very lucky to be in hospital at the time it happened. The trauma of this, of course, could have perhaps been avoided if I had been investigated seriously with my concerns. I kept seeing a different doctor every time. They could still see on their records that I had been in more than once and could have contacted the A and E department for their advice in this situation or whether to send me across—hindsight is a wonderful thing. I got a "sorry" from the hospital staff as I was waiting for the operation, but it was over my proceeding journey with endometriosis that I would experience time and time again how women are not heard or feel patronised by some gynaecologists who talk as if they know more about a woman's body through the textbooks and classes they attend than the women themselves living in them.

You may feel this is a little harsh, and of course I am not talking about the experiences of all women in medical settings, but this is how I've felt many times. It seems I am far from alone. I wondered if I was going crazy and if it was just me that felt that there was an injustice in how I was being dealt with. It felt like there were still hints in the medical setting of a historical era of eye watering ways in which women have been dealt with by doctors. The diagnosis of "hysteria" and "it's all in your head."

Science writer Abby Norman, who also has endometriosis, explains her own experience and research on this in her book, *Ask Me About My Uterus*. (You will find my thoughts on how we might have been taken away from some of our feminine wisdom in this book.)

I would later know all of this trauma to be the beginning of some beautiful discoveries, and the path towards a deeper calling.

It was after the emergency surgery and a few months of breastfeeding that my "period" returned. There was no blood, only extreme pain in my abdomen that had me in A and E. I did not know it was my period at the time, I had no idea what was wrong, and I was sent home with opiate painkillers as many women with endometriosis are.

This type of painkiller can cause constipation, which could potentially make the discomfort worse than it already is. I realised that it was happening every four weeks, so I felt it had to be related to my period, even though the pain was also around my stomach and navel area too and it continued for several months. What ensued were many hospital visits and anxiety around what was happening in my body, whilst desperately trying to look after a new baby and a one-year-old. I never really asked for help. Like many women, I felt I should be able to get on with things; after all, that's what women do, right?

That's what I'd witnessed many women in my life doing. I felt I needed to be strong, or what I assumed was strength at the time. Of course, strength would have been to show my vulnerability and ask for help. We must speak out, the large numbers of us who have endo (or other female conditions or traumas); silence does not beget change or awareness. By speaking out, we allow others to do the same, and when women gather in support, we can be a powerful force. It's hard to heal in your own silence.

With no bleeding and just extreme pain in my abdomen, I believed that after surgery to remove my placenta, my womb may have had some adhesions, resulting in a condition known as Asherman's syndrome, although this was never confirmed.

If I was bleeding, it wasn't able to leave my body and so I feel it could have caused retrograde menstruation which could have added to my already suspected endometriosis.

The theory of retrograde menstruation leading possibly to endometriosis was acknowledged by Dr. Sampson. The blood containing endometrial cells travels backwards into the fallopian tubes and pelvic area and stays there as a lesion (displaced/abnormal tissue). This is thought, however, to happen with many women when menstruating and whereas the immune system of many women's bodies clears it up, for some women, the cells remain outside the pelvis, and the hormonally sensitive tissue that is not where it should be follows the same cycle as the womb lining at menstruation. Bleeding into the pelvis when a woman menstruates, resulting in inflammation and pain.

However, retrograde menstruation does not explain why endometriosis lesions have been found in female foetuses. Or why some teenage girls have endometriosis (I will begin to refer intermittently to this condition as "endo") in their younger years or from the first cycle. Or that it has been found rarely in men. Also, the endo cells are said to be "like" the ones in the lining of the womb that react in the same way as the cells in the womb, building up and breaking down at menstruation.

It may be the case that for some women they are prone due to a number of factors to develop the disease later in life. I also had a tilted womb and found both of my boys breech until towards the end with both of my pregnancies. Luckily, my first turned eventually, but with my second, I was left with the option of ECV (manual turning of the baby) or C-section, and neither of those appealed to me. The shape of my pelvis and womb whilst menstruating, I believe, may have played a part in my endo. There were many other factors that I would later uncover that I feel added to menstrual pain.

For around seven months, I was in and out of hospital being prescribed painkillers and told to wait for my gynaecologist appointment at the BSGE centre (British Society for Gynaecological Endoscopy), or what are known as specialist endometriosis centres. There are a few of these dotted around the country. Once I was finally seen by an endo specialist, they could not see anything on the scan they provided and so I was referred to a gastroenterologist to check for a bowel problem before I would be offered the possibility of a laparoscopy (keyhole surgery). The trouble is, a scan can miss endo, which is why laparoscopy is the only way to diagnose it properly.

I was angry and frustrated. The pattern was around every four weeks and a specialist centre was sending me to a gastroenterologist, but I had classic endo symptoms and had it suspected prior to my births with an MRI that showed what looked like a large lesion in the pouch of douglas, the area between the rectum and the posterior wall of the womb.

This unfortunately is very common for women with endo, and diagnosis can take seven to ten years on average. A fire of injustice began to simmer within me; how could this be?

The more I discovered and experienced myself, the angrier I became. Why was women's healthcare being failed in so many ways? Not just for endo sufferers. I could write many books on women's health experiences and struggles to get necessary support, or to just be heard. This is also where it becomes important to empower and support ourselves.

In this day and age, how can we have a disease that affects one in ten women and has the potential to have such a dire consequence on the quality of life of those afflicted be so poorly researched and understood? Why had so few people heard of it?

If it affected both sexes, such as other diseases like Asthma or Crohn's or Celiac disease, would people know more about it? It still astonishes me how the public cannot know about such a devastating disease and the struggle women with endo go through to be heard or supported, let alone receive appropriate care. I realise that I speak from a position of privilege in the UK as there are some countries where the level of care for endometriosis is much worse or women cannot afford to pay for treatment. Endometriosis needs worldwide support.

I've heard enough stories from other women who also have been disregarded with their pain, made to feel like they are just "drama queens" because, hey, it can't really be that bad. There are so many women with endo who have stories about extreme pain and being sent home with advice to take a couple of paracetamols and use a hot water bottle, their doctors seriously displaying a lack of understanding about the toll endo can take. Never mind the many younger women who have been told they are "too young" to have endo. Some of the suffering comes from a lack of care, understanding or awareness of how debilitating it can be. You cannot see endo and scar tissue and the damage it is causing internally and pain is subjective so outwardly you can look fine. Women with endo are used to putting on a brave face when they are experiencing pain, possibly because it is so misunderstood that sometimes we give up trying to explain it. With more awareness and understanding this can change.

It is incredibly frustrating when little is known about the true cause of a disease. I am far from alone in feeling this. The science is not there yet as to why women develop endometriosis, although there are theories and speculations, one of which I've outlined. What we do know for certain is that the lesions are oestrogen sensitive.

The truth is there are so many questions with so few answers, there has not been the investment, interest or research into the disease from a medical point of view, this is a serious concern when you think about the research gone into other diseases. Trust me when I say, mine is just one story from many similar stories from other women with the disease and we are beginning to speak out. This book is about what I've discovered about it from an experiential perspective.

Doctors hand out various prescriptions, sometimes giving the impression that they are the authority on the best path for you. But if it's regarding menstrual conditions, it's always worth doing your own research and asking questions so you play a part in the decisions. Be assertive with what you feel you need but know that there are many women having success reducing or eliminating symptoms through holistic approaches too, this goes for all reproductive conditions. You may want or need both but make sure you are presented with all the risks and benefits to make an informed choice, whatever route you decide to take. Many doctors don't have the time that most of their patients need, and I do not envy the stress of their workloads. Most of them are genuinely trying to help in the way they know how, but the truth is, no one understands endo more than the women afflicted, especially when symptoms don't fall under the "classic symptoms".

Endometriosis can affect far more than the reproductive system; it has an impact on other systems like the nervous and immune systems. It has also been found in the lungs, nose and even the brain, although this is rare. But women do lose organs to endo. There is even more of a struggle in diagnosis for those who have it in other areas. I suspected endo in the thoracic area. I feel blessed that the disease didn't cause me too much difficulty in my younger years and to those whom it is affecting, there is hope and ways to support yourself that you may not have considered—this applies to many menstrual conditions too, as my experiences showed me.

My hormones were imbalanced, and my body began reacting to the disease in other ways. My immune system was low, and I ended up poorly with pneumonia (possibly related to suspected endo in the thoracic area) and back in hospital. My body couldn't cope with the stress of looking after two young children and a disease that was rapidly raging on the inside. It was a call from my body—if I wasn't going to slow down, I would be made to.

My heart goes out to any women suffering with illness whilst looking after children. I knew my body was desperately crying out for rest and a chance to rebalance and recover. The truth is, I could have put them in childcare at that point and focused on getting better, but I felt guilty and very sad that I might miss the baby phase. I was also lucky to even have it as an option in the first place. It was by far the most challenging and difficult year of my life. My body desperately needed to stop and recover, but there was no time; I had to keep going. Eventually I had no choice but to find another way. I was surviving and pushing through as much as I could, but I was becoming very unwell.

I tried desperately to get back to an endo centre after they sent me to a gastroenterologist to let them know I was certain I had endo or Asherman's as a result of what happened, or that it had aggravated existing disease. Unfortunately, it would take far too long, as they have long wait lists. And so, I ended up going back to the hospital that originally referred me to the specialist centre, sigh.

I managed to get a laparoscopy booked in for a few weeks after I had my consultation, and surprise, they found endo. The surgery was not carried out by an excision specialist, which is what I wanted. There is a difference between ablation (burning the surface whilst possibly leaving deeper disease) and excision (complete excision of disease tissue). Also, with ablation, the tissue is destroyed and so it cannot be sent to pathology to check on cancerous possibilities.

There are only a number of gynaecologists who are qualified in endometriosis advanced excision surgery in the UK and in other countries, so women might be at risk of receiving inadequate treatment, with disease left behind. Not the fault of the gynaecologist; they may not have been trained in the techniques and skills necessary for advanced disease. An excision specialist knows where and what to look for and will often work in a multidisciplinary team with a bowel or bladder surgeon. They will aim to eradicate deeper disease. Some endo lesions can unfortunately be very difficult to spot.

However, I was very grateful for that surgery as I bled again two weeks later for the first time in months, and the levels of pain had reduced. It gave me the respite I needed and some time to take charge of my health again.

Interestingly, on the follow-up appointment post-surgery, I was told that it was a coincidence I had bled again after the surgery. Hmmm, I thought, it may be because hospitals do not like to admit to Asherman's cases as it can be the outcome of surgery; it is not a disease of itself. I had already signed a form to accept the risk and possibility of Asherman's before the surgery, so it was not this in itself that was frustrating. It just seemed to be discounted immediately when I mentioned it. I had also read that Asherman's could be more likely following birth if women have had a 'D and C' for a retained placenta. This is because the womb is not yet healed properly. Perfectly logical, it was confusing because I couldn't believe how quickly it was discounted when I expressed my concerns that this is what could have been causing all the pain with no bleeding. It was the fact that it was dismissed out of hand with no investigation, and at this stage, I didn't have much energy to argue. I only wanted to get better so that I could look after my very young children. I will never know if this was truly the case.

There were many GPs and endo specialists who recommended the pill to me. It has helped with the management of symptoms for some women, providing relief, but others find they are eventually in worse pain or experience side effects, and it does not cure the disease. I was not looking for a suppression of symptoms. I also find it "intriguing" that women who only ovulate once a month are predominantly taking hormonal contraception, with many different options continually presenting themselves. Where are all the options regarding hormonal contraception for men? Ahem.

I had a strong intuitive sense that this was not the way forward that I wanted to take. I was not comfortable altering my already imbalanced hormonal system in this way. I felt that if my body was imbalanced or dis-eased, then I wanted to find a way to put the "ease" back in. I wanted to return to health and thought that there must be a way of using other natural methods to allow my body to restore itself. I wasn't looking for a magic pill, I wanted to return my body and hormones back to a state of balance so that it could be in a stronger position to heal itself, or at least reduce inflammation and other symptoms.

Again, upon reflection, this was all part of my journey. I could never bring myself to take the pill at any time in my life and I wasn't sure why I felt so strongly about it, but my intuition said no. I was also a reflexologist at the time and knew there were lots of holistic ways to help myself. I was about to make some beautiful discoveries about menstruation, so this intuitive sense seems very "coincidental" considering what later transpired.

I was also, however, very aware that the D and C for my retained placenta had caused a lot of damage in my pelvic area and that I would not rule out another surgery. I was very clear that if I ever needed surgery again that I would have an endo surgeon I could trust and who would be qualified in excision surgery.

I began my research and decided to have a private consultation with a surgeon in Birmingham who was renowned for his expertise but also for listening to his patients.

His clinic had a good atmosphere, and I felt at ease upon meeting my surgeon. He had a warm and welcoming smile and a presence or air about him that I instinctively felt trusting towards. Even my husband commented on his presence without me saying anything about how I felt, which made me smile. For the first time, I felt as if I had been listened to with empathy. He had the same frustration I did, having heard many times from other women how difficult it was to get diagnosed and receive appropriate care. I knew straight away that if I needed surgery again, it would be with him. I was aware that the surgery I had received previously would not have removed all my disease and that the surgeon had not checked the bowel and all other areas that endometriosis can hide. He had also ablated and not excised.

We made the decision that we would leave it a few months before deciding whether to go ahead with excision surgery. This was because my symptoms had improved from the previous laparoscopy. And now that I was bleeding again and had some lesions destroyed, I had some relief. I didn't want surgery again at that time. I wanted to see what I could do to improve any lingering symptoms or stop the development of any further disease.

Every time we met for our follow-up appointments, I delayed, as my symptoms had reduced drastically after following the methods and insights laid out in this book. But I still had the sense that he was at some point going to help me or be part of my unfolding story. I also had a fear that I would end up in a situation like before, not getting the treatment I needed. I was still anxious after not being heard so many times. My body was still on high alert after so much trauma. I did not know then what I know now.

The support began as I ventured on my quest to return my health on all levels. I was about to unpeel so much wisdom that I had no idea I could access. Magical and mysterious synchronicities began to occur in my life, which led me here, over two years later, to write this book now.

I ask you to question your own feelings around what your menstrual cycle or womb means to you. Whether positive or negative associations or even nothing, write it down on paper, especially if it represents anger, pain or frustration. You can keep checking back in to see if your associations or feelings change.

If you do suffer from endometriosis or any reproductive issues, or if you are just looking to connect to your body with wisdom and love through self-care, this book offers a truly holistic and empowering feminine path. I hope the methods and insights I discovered could give you the same joy, wisdom, feminine reconnection and respite they gave me.

BUT FIRST, WE NEED TO SPEAK OUT ABOUT PERIODS!!

PART OF THE problem for women with gynaecological conditions is a feeling of shame around discussing menstrual health. Why is this? It's worth reflecting on a history of women's voices being silenced.

With past suspicions of women (think witch burnings) and even in cultures still today, women have been asked to leave whilst on their periods because it is considered dirty or suspicious. It has been made a taboo subject to talk about.

The more we speak out, the easier it will be for others who are currently suffering alone.

There is some change happening and a greater recognition and awareness of conditions such as endo, fibroids, and polycystic ovarian syndrome which are all beginning to be aired more regularly in the media and are gaining some traction with research, but why has it taken so long? I know many of us with endo are used to looking at the confused faces of others when we tell them we are suffering with the disease.

Endometriosis and other menstrual conditions need a voice and so do our various routes to self-care and an understanding of our innate feminine cyclical wisdom. Why the shame? If you feel it and cannot say when you are on your period, ask yourself, where does this shame come from? What am I in fear of? What is causing me to feel shame when it is a natural part of being a woman and without our menstrual blood, we wouldn't have the human race, I mean seriously, huh? Let's investigate this relationship between our female bodies and our cycles, especially the amount of pain experienced by many.

The more discussions we have regarding menstrual health, the easier it will be for others to identify issues and eradicate shame. More importantly, we can discuss how these conditions might not manifest in the first place, or they can be helped, and symptoms reduced or even possibly eliminated if they do. And even further than this, see how much of a gift our cycle can be. Stay with me.

Many women are suffering whether they are on their periods or menopausal. Thankfully, awareness is increasing as women start to speak out about the menopause too, discussing how it is affecting them physically and in their psyche. There would be far less fear and confusion if the education was there on ways to support each other on how to navigate the changing landscape, both from physical symptoms and with the psycho-spiritual and archetypal changes, which this book will discuss. It's amazing how fear and confusion can turn into love and acceptance, including a bunch of gifts that can arise throughout the process.

Examples of inappropriate messages sent to women regarding their periods include some of the adverts that have been broadcast for menstrual products. Often showing women being active in some way or wearing white or tight shorts or leggings.

The connotations being that if we use their products we will feel great, not leak blood and can "continue on as normal with our lives". Who is creating these adverts?

I feel that is not what most women want to be doing when on our periods. I would much rather be curled up with chocolate and a good film. What message are we sending to many women who feel far from that at menstruation? I'll stick with comfy underwear, thanks. Our energy often does ask us to rest at this phase and take up methods of self-care that allow us to recharge and let go of that which needs releasing; more on this later.

FERTILITY/WOMB MASSAGE

MY MISSION TO understand and empower myself with endo began unexpectedly one year after I had the postnatal operation and severe endo pain. As a reflexologist at the time, I was receiving a lot of fertility clients and I heard about fertility massage (www.fertilitymassage.co.uk) developed by the wonderful Clare Spink. I read online about her course and it sounded great, especially the fact that it would be experiential for us as therapists too. It is important to acknowledge that it can be used for all women, particularly for those of us with menstrual conditions, not just for fertility.

The training ran over a period of four days, and the course I attended was in February. It was cold, and I was still experiencing some symptoms and fatigue from everything that had happened the previous year. It was only about two to three months since I had been poorly with pneumonia and I was tired from my body having been so unwell the year before and from looking after my boys. I was hoping I had the energy to go to London to attend the training course. I remember feeling a strong desire to go, but I wasn't sure why at the time, my eldest child was feeling a little poorly and I felt guilty for leaving him.

When we arrived, we sat in circle and we were asked to express how we were feeling in that exact moment. Not having to put on a social front, we were encouraged to feel into our truth, whatever that was. It sounds so simple and it is, but it was amazing how many of us felt so vulnerable to speak it. We are so used to saying "I'm fine" so as not to break the peace or make someone feel uncomfortable or unsettle them. It felt like a long time since I'd felt vulnerable, probably because we don't often meet people for such a short period of time and express our honest truths and feelings. But as others started to express theirs, we all began to open up.

As a group of women, we were beginning to trust that it was ok to share our truths, something that many of us felt was new. Most the time, we try to hide or not express our true emotions for fear of how we will be perceived or judged, as already mentioned, and so we were wary at first to be so open.

It was whilst writing about this that I came across this quote from Parker J. Palmer who is a columnist at On Being (onbeing. org) from his article, "*The Gift of Presence, The Perils of Advice.*" He argues:

"Here's the deal. The human soul doesn't want to be advised or fixed or saved. It simply wants to be witnessed—to be seen, heard and companioned exactly as it is. When we make that kind of deep bow to the soul of a suffering person, our respect reinforces the soul's healing resources, the only resources that can help the sufferer make it through."

I noticed the synchronicity of finding this quote and it describes perfectly what happened to us all as we sat in circle daily on our training. We were being truly witnessed, seen and heard, warts and all. It was a revelation for all of us to be held in such a supportive space. To feel that we could be safe in being truly honest, even with ourselves, and to feel the power held energetically in that circle. It felt good not to be given advice, or to be told how we could change our circumstances; we were being validated in our truth in that moment. Next time someone tries to advise you with your struggles, see how it would feel if you told them that you didn't want advice, that you just want to be acknowledged as you are in that moment. And do the same in return for others. Your soul and theirs will appreciate it.

It was as if something within me had woken up whilst on this training course. It was so much more than I expected. It was a retreat with knowledge that I had no idea I needed. And it was the first time in a while where I had felt that feeling that I was exactly where I was supposed to be. It was mysterious in the timing of it as I thought I was just going on a course to add a therapy to my practice. I had no idea it was exactly what I needed at that precise time myself.

Throughout the course, we were experiencing the therapy as well as treating each other and so we were going through our own healing process. I felt surges of energy both in and after the course. This energy can be described as the Shakti energy (related to the feminine energy force) rising, and it felt as though my body and its senses were waking up from a deep sleep. After a year of struggle and survival, I truly felt a shift. It was the start of my journey to emotional, spiritual and physical healing.

We journeyed through visualisations, connecting to the womb and pelvic bowl, seeing what insights would emerge through visual symbols or our emotions. The massage itself was the most beautiful, nurturing and spiritual treatment I had ever received. It seemed natural yet essential somehow, but it was also transformative in my experience and I have seen this with many of my clients too. It took a couple of days, but I finally began to release some of the trauma of the year post my second birth and proceeding endo struggle. Suppressed issues and emotional pain from my past seemed to arise from my subconscious. Most of us felt an awakening of wisdom, or what could be described as 'remembering', with this work. I began operating with a new awareness and deeper truths revealed themselves to me as a knowing from within. I was far more in touch with my feminine side and accessing my intuition.

When first being worked on myself, I felt really tense. With everything that had happened, my pelvis and reproductive system had become an area that I feared. It had caused me severe pain and I could have died from my haemorrhaging womb and so I was still holding a lot of trauma in this space. The nurturing touch was a revelation. I was surprised by how my body received it. Especially as I was wincing at the thought of the area being touched.

The body holds the wisdom, sensuality and intuition. The mind is often set to mute whilst receiving this therapy, allowing the soul voice to be heard. Most of us are living in our heads and have forgotten the energetic power and wisdom of our bodies. The course helped me identify ancestral patterns. Issues and genetics held in our DNA or energetically passed through. Remember that you were in your grandma! Your mum was carrying you in her eggs as a baby in your grandma's womb and so cycles and patterns can continue in families.

On a physical level, the womb massage aims to help remove old and stagnant blood and revitalise fresh blood to the area. I felt the massage helped to reposition my already tilted womb. It also aims to loosen adhesions and increase circulation and lymph flow in the area. There are contraindications to receiving this therapy which a trained fertility massage therapist will address, if you decide you want to try it. Especially do not massage if you have a coil inserted. The massage is so gentle and also works in conjunction with the digestive system in a clockwise direction to also aid any digestive issues.

After discussing whether it is safe for you with a practitioner, you can also do your own self-care massage using gentle strokes in a clockwise direction from your hip, across and above your navel and stroking down where the descending colon is, as well as small circles from hip to hip across the womb. Notice how you feel, what arises? I use organic coconut oil whilst massaging. Also set a relaxing space, you could have dimmed lights, music and essential oils in a diffuser. Tune into your emotional state and how you are feeling. Where do you feel your emotion in your body? Is it the chest? Or the stomach? Just feel without attaching any stories.

The abdomen and pelvis are usually areas that are untouched by massage, which can also be the case sometimes with pregnancy massage, and it is an area that can make women feel very vulnerable if they have menstrual conditions or previous traumas. With the mind/body connection, do you send love or anger to the area? I was definitely sending anger and frustration to mine for the destruction it was causing, rather than thinking about how I could ask what it was I needed or what changes I needed to make that would help me. I needed to be kinder to myself with what I was experiencing. How kind are you to yourself when you have pain? Do you feel angry and as though your body has turned against you? This is all worth enquiring about.

A common experience that also arises or is remembered with this treatment is saying yes at some stage to sexual encounters when we haven't wanted them; this is giving our power away. There is a chance that we then store the experience or push it down, turning it inwards and manifesting as misguided shame.

There are the physical benefits of the treatment, but also spiritual and emotional. When we begin to awaken to the energy of our womb space and heal our unmet needs or past traumas, it is possible to reawaken a sense of flow with life, especially if you are feeling stuck. Releasing any trauma or emotion that has been hidden away and blocked can cause subconscious patterns that will often play out in our lives. When you find the root cause of a belief that has stemmed from a past experience, it can no longer drive you without your awareness. You can begin to unlock outdated patterns and create change.

An example of hidden issues that can arise with women in my treatment room stem from emotional abuse or unmet needs by their parents when they were little. These are the very people they relied upon and encountered in their first experiences of love, and, of course, we are all dependant as children and in the process of forming belief systems. Through understanding hidden pain and misguided beliefs, self-love and learning to mother oneself can break disempowering patterns; journaling or caring for the inner child who may still be hurting. When we are constantly looking on the outside for love that we need to give to ourselves, we are giving our power away. Learning to empower and love yourself does not mean that others will not hurt you but that you can learn to soothe yourself and know that you have a strong core. You can begin to see where you are searching to fill a hole or the discomfort felt within by looking in the wrong place outside yourself. Self-love and mothering ourselves can often feel strange as a concept and many women will feel guilty about putting themselves first when society tells us that this is selfish. We need love and connection with others too, of course, but question how much you give to yourself. Do you speak differently to others, giving them good advice but not offering the same to yourself? Treat yourself as you would your best friend.

Most of us haven't given much love towards ourselves or our bodies throughout our lives, especially the womb area. If anything, we can take the frustration out on ourselves at the challenges of being female in a world that often doesn't respect cyclical needs, pushing when we need to rest, not eating when hungry or not sleeping enough and working too hard to obtain an ideal notion of "success" or squeezing ourselves into moulds that don't fit. This can also affect our health and menstrual cycle. If we don't respect our body and mental health, who will?

Putting how this treatment affected me personally into words is difficult as it is an embodied experience, and the way it affects everyone will be different, depending on your needs at the time. It is like a ritual, especially with the use of rebozos (traditional Mexican shawls) at the end.

Ritual was something else that I really began to benefit from in my own life. Many people, including psychologists, have discovered and researched the benefits of ritual and the power behind setting an intention. They can help you to focus on what you want. Whilst also helping you to be present in the moment. Ritual can help you to honour yourself and others in a spiritual and sacred way. They also help to connect to gratitude and appreciation and have been shown to reduce anxiety. Many cultures practice daily rituals together.

My body and psyche responded to this therapy in a way that astounded me. A loving feminine healing practice connecting to my womb in a way I never had before. I felt my period after the course as a release of some of the emotion and trauma from the previous year. It shifted my energy and I truly felt an ease of flow with my period for the first time in what felt like ages. It seemed magical.

This therapy and course supported and held me in a way that allowed me to begin processing the postnatal and endo experiences.

We also learnt about menstrual cycle awareness, this was where my understanding of my female body and feminine energies increased and I began to understand why I may have felt these physical, emotional and energetic shifts through working in this way. Revealing much wisdom. (More on this later).

The link of mind, body, and spirit was becoming very real. I was hungry to learn more, and the teachers began to show up.

RED TENT/ WOMEN'S CIRCLES

I WANTED TO find out more about women's circles after training with Clare. There is a resurgence of women's circles, or red tents, happening at the moment, sparked by the book, *The Red Tent* by Anita Diamont. A monthly space where women can show up exactly as they are, all emotions welcome. When you honour all your feelings, you are honouring yourself in the moment. Feelings when felt will move through and transform; hiding them means you might be trying to run away from a message your body might be giving you. You also risk becoming numb from all feelings when you try to avoid some. Is there any part of you that you are rejecting?

In a circle there is an option to just be in a space with other women, to reflect, journal, read, or just rest and retreat. There is often a creative element or sometimes dance but everyone who attends is free to do as they feel and is not obliged to participate in any facilitated activities. You can set up your own circle. Most start with a circle share as we did on our training. You can include essential oil diffusers, beautiful affirmations or cards to set the scene, chocolate always works! You might want to include beautiful fabrics to decorate the space and bring food to be shared. It's important to set an intention for the group and make sure that everyone understands they have a certain amount of time (usually two to three minutes) to share in the circle. The others are to listen, rather than try to fix things. This holds a container for the group so that it follows a structure for the energy to work within rather than going off on tangents.

If hosting a red tent, decorate with red fabric, pillows and as much red as possible! This is the colour of blood and power, representing the menstrual cycle. It can be a revelation to honour rather than abhor our cycle. I spent a lot of time frustrated and annoyed by my cycle. I now see that instead of supporting or honouring my body and its messages, I was fighting against it and raging at it, hurting myself further in the process. I was increasing stress, which is the worst thing you can do with an inflammatory disease. This creates a response with the adrenals, releasing cortisol, but when this reaction occurs, too often it's going to impact the immune and other systems that might be struggling already under health conditions such as endo. This can cause further hormonal imbalance in the long run so always see what you can do to reduce stress in your life. I found women's circles were great for stress release.

The red tents of the past were a place where women would go to bleed and recuperate, bringing back wisdom to their communities. It was acknowledged that many women's cycles would sync with the moon and many women would bleed together. Women who were not bleeding would come and support women who were with massage and food, conversation, and ceremony.

Native Americans in the past had lodges set up for women to retreat to whilst menstruating, but rather than viewed as shameful or derogatory, women were revered when bleeding. There would be ritual and ceremony. The fact that women could bleed without dying was a mysterious and amazing concept and seen as a purification process, a renewal.

You could also set up or attend a moon lodge, where women meet on the new or full moon to do a ritual release or set intentions for the coming moon cycle. There could be meditation and some creative activity similar to women's circles.

MENSTRUAL AND LUNAR CYCLES, THE GIFT OF MENSTRUATION.

(YEP, I SAID GIFT, AND I HAVE ENDO! I AM SURPRISED I COULD SAY THIS TOO.)

THERE IS SO much more to your menstrual cycle than you may have realised. There is the obvious, that we are able to create babies, but it can also mean so much more. Each cycle can be a guide to our creativity and inner power whilst prompting our needs and our directions in life. I began experiencing my own cycle, eventually, as an inner gift, using it like an inbuilt mindfulness practice for women. For someone with endo or other menstrual issues, this could be difficult to understand if it is only causing grief and pain, and I can totally empathize. But if you can, there is a chance that you can work with your cycle to gain wisdom from it. If in the depths of pain or disease consider taking the full holistic approach with other methods discussed in the book, especially the nutrition section and the importance of a healthy digestive system. Only you will know if you need or want medical care, too. Empowerment comes through feeling that you are making the right choices for you regardless of the opinions of other's. These methods of self-care can support us whatever decisions we take. Let's delve into how working with the cycle could support you.

I gained knowledge and wisdom from a number of menstrual cycle awareness authors, leaders and teachers, such as: Alexandra Pope and Sjanie Hugo Wurlitzer *(Wild Power)*, Lisa Lister *(Code Red)* and Miranda Gray *(Red Moon)*. I attended Menstrual Medicine Circle (a unique process developed by Alexandra Pope and Sjanie Hugo Wurlitzer) with Leora Leboff. A beautiful, wise woman who has witnessed my journey from the start. It was through my training in fertility massage with the wonderful Clare Spink that I initially discovered the power of womb connection and cycle awareness. I used many tools on the path to healing and gaining wisdom from my own cycle, specifically to find relief from postnatal surgery and endometriosis.

As women, most of us have lost touch with our natural rhythms through living for the most part in a patriarchal society where energy is linear—go, go, go, work, work, work, without much emphasis on rest and recuperation. Not even thinking about leisure time or just time out to do something that gives us pleasure, just because we want to. It's interesting to hear how many people say they feel guilty about this. I think it should be a necessity. Life is too short to not make time to enjoy it, and it is often our societies' pressures that stop us from remembering this.

So, when women have their menstrual cycle, this by nature is a time that we may want to rest and retreat inwards. In many cultures, this might happen, but for most of us, we are striving and pushing on regardless of our bodies' callings.

If we followed our cyclical rhythms and were able to live more in tune with our cycle and offer the necessary self-care we need, as I discovered, there is an opportunity to reduce or eliminate menstrual pain and increase joy. Even finding our calling in life or connecting to our inner feminine wisdom.

I began to think about the different energies within us, such as yang (masculine) and yin (feminine), and how we all, both men and women, have a combination of both. The idea from the Tao is that in nature we have a balance of the two and that despite being opposite, they are interdependent on each other. Our culture and society tend to praise the masculine/yang way of "doing" and outer manifestation rather than the yin/feminine way of "being" and our inner world, creating imbalances and issues in our bodies and lives.

Yang/Masculine energy is more outer-focused, analytical, logical, linear, task-orientated, competitive and involved with activities and manifestation in the world, and giving out our energy. It is related to the sun, light, and daytime. Interestingly, it is said to be related to the right side of the body. Many of my symptoms and endo was found on the right side. I was certainly dominant in this energy and it seems the imbalance may have played out physically on this side of my body. As if my body was telling me that I needed to investigate this. It often came up in healing sessions.

Yin energy, its opposite, represents the "being" rather than "doing" aspect of ourselves: receptive, receiving, intuitive, collaborative and restoring. Relating to night, darkness and the moon and the left side of the body. We know which one is deemed as more important in our cultures.

Some of us will by nature resonate more with one of these energies. In my own life I feel I resonated very much with yang and outer energy and expression but forgot the importance of yin. When I began to address both within myself and started acknowledging the shifts in my menstrual cycle and psyche, I could feel into the yin energy and I found I reconnected to my intuition and could see many benefits of "receiving" and "being" rather than "doing" that helped with reducing any symptoms caused by endo. It was revelatory to me that a disease that was affecting my female reproductive system was helped by connecting to the feminine/yin energy, recognising the need to restore a balance. It is often difficult at first to connect to this yin/feminine energy as we may have been made to feel that we are "useless" or "unloveable" if we don't achieve or manifest something by doing.

We live in a time where, for so many of us, we struggle to get the space or time we need to rest. But just being present and having the awareness of your cyclic nature as a woman, offering yourself the smallest self-care, such as time out for a cup of coffee or a bath, and connecting in to your internal state can be enough. I found it transformative to do menstrual cycle awareness and I hope you will, too.

To start, we will look at the different energies present in a woman's cycle and how I experienced my own cycle in each phase. Just like the seasons of nature, we follow similar patterns in our own cyclic process, with the rise and fall in hormones.

If you no longer have a cycle as you have completed menopause or had a hysterectomy, you can follow the same guidance you might receive from the menstrual cycle, but instead, tracking the moon and its phases to use this as a cyclical guide. Menopause itself will hold its own process and inherent wisdom.

The moon follows a cycle through phases as seen from our perspective on earth. We can see the moon at night due to the reflection of the sun. It completes its orbit from one new moon to the next around every twenty-nine and a half days. It has a time frame similar to the menstrual cycle, between day one of menstruation and then through the cycle and back again. Coincidence?

Many others throughout history and in the present have followed the phases of the moon with rituals and practices. Gardeners have been known to plant crops via the moon phases.

So how could all this relate to us?

We are cyclical and just like the tides we could be affected by the moon, and we are affected by our menstrual cycle.

Note: If you have any menstrual conditions or endo, see if you can tune into any feelings or issues that might arise with the pain. Up the self-care as much as you can and consider incorporating the full holistic approach as mentioned previously. I discuss in the second half of this book the other approaches I took. I had some incredible insights and experienced menstruation in a completely different way through charting my cycle whilst using a combination of healing modalities. I reduced my symptoms and was able to really experience these shifts in my psyche and changing needs as outlined below.

Linking the seasons to our menstrual cycle:

- **Winter season linked to menstruation.**
- **Spring season linked to pre-ovulation.**
- **Summer season linked to ovulation.**
- **Autumn season linked to post ovulation.**

WINTER - MENSTRUATION

WINTER IN NATURE is when the trees are barren, and everything has retreated. It is the time in our menstrual cycle where we are bleeding and wanting the outside pressures to fall away, naturally releasing and retreating inwards ourselves if we are lucky.

There is often a deepening of inner wisdom felt in this phase of our cycles if you take time to connect with yourself and listen. It is a time when our bodies naturally want us to stop.

If you can, try not to book important meetings or presentations. This will not fit into your energy and needs at this stage of your cycle and you may feel resentful. If it is not possible, just acknowledge that and then let it go; the awareness can help you move through with more ease.

It can be a great time to catch up on a book or to do some journaling. I found journaling helped bring forth insights and I was able to integrate the lessons. The energy in this part of the cycle is inwards—containing, healing and intuitive, a perfect time for a ritual release around anything that no longer serves us.

Menstruation is also a great time to let any emotional baggage you are carrying go. I once burned from my journal an issue

I wanted to release from my life and my bleed came straight away. Feeling very connected to the wisdom of the body and psyche as the bleed is about releasing.

Sleep well and go to bed early if you can. You can also decode your dreams as they can be more vivid when menstruating. Often with self-care and rest you will awaken to the next phase of spring (pre-ovulation) with enthusiasm and space to create anew. Whatever you have let go of or released will not need to come with you into the next phase of your cycle. It can be easier to accept what has happened in your past if it is still affecting you in the present. Integrate any lessons, wisdom or strength gained from your experiences in order to move forwards. Open up to the uncertainty of the future, feel into what wants to come through you. Any inspirations? Are you being called towards something? Listen to this.

The winter/menstruation phase is also the time when ideas are being incubated underground. It is not time for them to come out into the light yet. Nurture your ideas, water them like seeds waiting to grow. Give them what they need before they will grow into the light (spring).

As you retreat into yourself, you can imagine being co-cooned in a cave. If you are working or busy, you can visualise that you are protected in your cave. It will be a time for renewal. If you have a flexible working schedule or are able to work from home, then this is the best time to do so. Also try and book in some time for yourself. Let everything in your life settle and if possible, try not to push or strive for anything.

The biggest gift that the winter stage of my menstrual cycle gave me was the importance of setting boundaries. You must be truthful with your 'no's and prioritise what matters. I began to really see how not taking time out for self-care at this stage of my cycle would affect the next stage and even the rest of my cycle. We all have these shifts in our menstrual cycles, but I'd never really taken note before. I would always be trying to do too much in the winter phase and naturally we feel more tired as we bleed, more frustrated by the demands of the outside world. Many women will find having children at this phase of the cycle more difficult. This is because children can be demanding, and I often found it challenging because I had increased my awareness of what my body needed at this time, but I wasn't always able to give myself what I needed. This is true for all of us at times. I found that the acceptance of my situation, and surrendering to it, with a few deep breaths, helped clear the frustration. If I could catch a bath or even take five to ten minutes to read, it helped me reset. It was a tool of self-care. I found my senses were heightened in this phase and I would receive clear signals and messages about what needed changing in my life.

In the autumn/winter phase of the cycle, I found that I felt guilty about working or would feel sad if I had not had much quality time with my children. This is an example of the kind of issues that may arise and need addressing.

Up the self-care by taking walks or anything that helps you retreat from the outside world. This is the phase I love going to the cinema and watching a good film. Book a massage. It is a great time to have a ritual bath, putting in some of your favourite essential oils, taking a herbal tea, or glass of champagne. (Your preference; mine is always chocolate!) Set the intention to rest and let go. Wear your comfy clothes or pyjamas if at home.

Related energetically to the Dark Moon (we cannot see the moon from earth)

Also linked to the New Moon (we start to see a small part of the moon)

Linked to the Crone archetype.

TCM (Traditional Chinese Medicine)—Links to yin energy.

The pituitary gland starts producing LH (Luteinising hormone) and FSH (Follicle Stimulating Hormone) to stimulate the growth of new follicles (for egg development). Progesterone and oestrogen are at their lowest, and this can affect your happy hormones. More so if you're stressed and not eating well.

Meditation on Winter—What does your winter scene look like at this stage of your cycle? Close your eyes, one hand on heart and one on the womb, gentle music in the background. Connect into the pelvic bowl and wait for visuals to come to you. You can walk a path to your womb temple. What does the path look like? Does anyone meet you at the temple? Do they have any messages for you? How does your womb temple make you feel?

Journal, draw or paint the scene.

Support with stretching exercise or going for gentle walks. Most women will crave meat for B vitamins and iron in this phase to replace what is lost through their bleed. With endo I started out as vegan on supplements and then eventually added small amounts of grass-fed organic meat to avoid animals that may have been fed antibiotics or a diet involving pesticides. Talk to a nutritionist to make a plan for your cycle. Make sure you eat vitamin C rich foods to help with iron absorption. Connect in to what you feel your body needs.

SPRING - PRE-OVULATION

PRE-OVULATION IS LIKE our inner spring, where everything begins to blossom. So with this stage of our cycle, we are coming out of menstruation and beginning to feel a rise in our energy levels as oestrogen rises again. We become physically stronger, new ideas and creative projects begin to emerge, just like new buds are sprouting from the ground in nature.

This has always been one of my favourite times of the year and of my menstrual cycle. I am sure there is no coincidence in this as they offer the same energy. (It also used to mean that I was passed the pain of menstruation!) In nature, the seed's potential and growth is beginning to manifest in the world. We start to see the green shoots. The energy is moving and starting to express itself, full of excitement and potential, and it can be the same for us at this stage of our cycle. We start to take hold of the insights and ideas that were brewing in menstruation/winter and give them expression to the outside world.

I have been known to be "enthusiastic" and I love the feeling at this stage of my cycle. There is youth and vitality present, but we must be careful not to run forth with our ideas and creations as they still need nurturing to a completion. If I was to send this book out with the enthusiasm of this stage without having it scrutinised or edited or refined, it would likely have mistakes, and wouldn't be complete. If ideas came to light during the winter phase of menstruation, this is the time to decide what to do with those ideas; how to use them and whether or when to use them. It could be like a premature birth; as excited as you are to meet your baby, you want them to incubate and grow to a healthy size before meeting them. It is the same for your creative projects. Allow the energy of this time in your cycle to settle.

I find I like to wear brighter clothes to express myself in this phase, and I like to be more experimental with food. Cooking for others feels more enjoyable. You might find your confidence levels increase and you feel lightness and joy. I also discovered that I can get scattered due to the dynamic energy that can be present in this phase. I have needed to rein myself in regularly, but I find making lists and planning comes more naturally to me here, particularly with regard to business ideas or projects. Your memory improves as this may have been affected in menstruation when hormone levels drop.

Related energetically to the Waxing Moon Phase (we can see more of the moon daily)

Linked to the Maiden archetype.

TCM—Linked to yin energy.

The womb lining thickens and grows. One of the many follicles produced at menstruation becomes dominant,

producing more oestrogen. This increase in oestrogen starts to inhibit the secretion of FSH which means that the smaller follicles start to die off as they are left to "starve" of FSH.

Meditation on Spring—Sit with eyes closed and some gentle background music, one hand on heart, one hand on womb, and connect into the pelvic bowl. What visual arises for you here? Is the area hot or cold? What can you see in your pelvic bowl? Is the texture rough or smooth? When you connect to your ovaries, how are they looking? What visuals might represent your ovaries? Chains? Flowers? Colours?

After this, you can draw the scene of your springtime. When I do this exercise in this part of my cycle, I often see the sun and space around me with a lot of colour and warmth. This is often a representation of how I feel in this part of my cycle.

Exercise might start to get easier as you head towards ovulation. Support with leafy greens, eggs and fish (if not affected by eggs or fish) to help with the growth of the womb lining and continue support after the blood loss of menstruation. If looking to conceive, then consider increasing immune supporting foods to help with the implantation of the egg.

SUMMER – OVULATION

OVULATION IS LIKE our inner summer, when our energy is at its peak and our ideas are starting to manifest. Creativity is enhanced, and creative ideas can come to fruition in this phase, as the plans we made in spring are manifesting. We can be on a high with life!

In nature, the sun is out, and many flowers are in full bloom, and there is high energy. This phase of our menstrual cycle relates to the Mother archetype; it is a nurturing, loving and giving time.

You may find it easier to be selfless, whether that is with children, pets, community or charity projects. I love this phase with my children. I have more energy to run around with them, and it is a great time to plan or to have a holiday with them. I find I do not get as easily stressed by the demands of having small children in this phase.

It's also easier to concentrate, channel and focus on projects and desires. We may glow in radiance. You may feel your sexual energy and attraction peaks around ovulation because it is the time of conception, if trying for a baby. However, our sexual energy does not need to be used for sex; it can be used for our projects.

We may feel at ease and in flow with life and are able to tap into what is working for us.

Work-wise, it is a great time for planning important meetings and projects. We can find it easier to be compassionate with ourselves and others, more open and receptive as our energy is radiating outwards.

It's a great time to be social and plan for social events as the energy and enthusiasm flows. You want to get out and meet friends. It is also the best time to meet new people and attend groups or courses that interest you.

Your life can feel abundant.

Related energetically to the Full Moon (we can see all of the moon illuminated)

Linked to the Mother archetype.

TCM—Linked to yang energy.

When the level of oestrogen is high enough, it produces a surge of LH hormone which triggers the release of the egg from the dominant follicle.

Meditation on Summer—One hand on heart, one hand on womb. Connect into the space. How does it feel? What does it look like? If your womb was a plant, flower or tree, which one would it be?

Journal or draw what comes up for you in your summer scene and document whether there are any messages for you.

Support with all forms of exercise that interest you. Personally, I love dancing or yoga at this stage of my cycle. Foods rich in vitamin B and zinc are said to help with egg release and implantation if trying to conceive. Legumes could be supportive if vegan or vegetarian.

AUTUMN – POST-OVULATION

AUTUMN IS A time in nature when the leaves on the trees are falling away and in this phase of our menstrual cycle what needs to fall away in our lives will make itself known. It will become conscious in our feelings and psyche. Let what wants to fall away, fall. A rise in progesterone occurs and we may want to slow down, slinging out the old and anything that isn't working.

This is the phase that many women dread because it is a time when premenstrual tension can be present. But I began to see this phase as a gift. Suppressed emotions would bubble up to be acknowledged and worked with. If we have given our power away, we will find issue around that. Frustration at patriarchy or society's demands may unleash! Burn that shame!

It is usually in this phase when things that have been bothering you at other easier phases of your cycle will be aired. If, for example, you live with someone who doesn't empty the dishwasher, you may let this go in spring or summer when hormonally and energetically things are easier. But in autumn, it is time to speak the truth, and there is no filter to stop you as there might be in the other phases. Anything that isn't serving you will come to the fore. It can be a time for transformation and an acknowledgement of our shadow side. We may have to face reality if we are putting the veil of illusion over areas of our lives.

Bad relationship? It may become conscious and apparent. I found I sometimes shocked myself in this phase with what I discovered was no longer working for me. If writing a book, this stage of the cycle is perfect for scrutiny and editing. This applies to any area of our lives or projects that need it.

It can be a difficult but rewarding phase if we listen to the messages but be wary not to get too attached if your inner critic is making life difficult.

I am not one for routine or mundane day-to-day activities and this is strong for me at this phase in the cycle as the previously tolerable becomes intolerable. It can be difficult with your children if they are being challenging, and we may not have the patience for it like we would in our summer phase. I found in the second half of my cycle that I wanted more alone time. You will find that if you haven't taken care of your needs at other times in your cycle this phase could be more challenging.

I felt my senses were heightened and I was connected to my intuition; psychic abilities were stronger. I found I could connect more intuitively into my clients' needs.

It is important in this phase to up the self-care. This includes good nutritional intake. You are heading towards menstruation, and so make sure that hormonally you keep balanced. It certainly helps if you are feeling PMT. Make good nutritional choices, create time for self-care and love. We will probably find the inner critic is stronger. Let the inner critic be heard but be wary that you do not start attacking yourself or even believing the voice if it doesn't hold wisdom for you. Listen to the messages if they do hold a truth you need to hear, but ensure kindness to yourself, too.

Let what is no longer serving you be released through ritual or journaling, continuing into the winter phase.

Related energetically to the Waning Moon (We see less of the moon as the days go on)

Linked to the Enchantress archetype.

TCM—Linked to yang energy.

The follicle that released the egg is now called the corpus luteum. This produces progesterone. If pregnancy occurs, the progesterone stays until around ten weeks of gestation. The body's temperature can rise. If there is no conception, then progesterone eventually declines with the breakdown of the corpus luteum and the shedding of the lining at menstruation.

Meditation on Autumn—One hand on heart and one hand on womb. Connect into pelvic space. What does the area feel and look like in this phase of your cycle? Sit inside the cave of your womb. You see a scroll. What messages do you receive? What do you need to know?

Journal or draw the scene.

Support with exercise that feels good and releases endorphins, try not to push yourself in this phase. Warm comforting

foods such as soups, lentils and legumes are said to be good. Slow releasing carbohydrates are better to help with the hormonal shifts and to maintain blood sugar levels. Helping to keep your hormones steady.

The cycle continues again with menstruation, or if using the moon as a cyclic guide then back to the dark moon.

If you are dealing with any menstrual conditions or having trouble conceiving, you can consider a qualified nutritional therapist to support you. I include a section later on how I focused on anti-inflammatory and plant-based foods to help me for my endo.

Above is just a guide to the energy usually dominant in each phase of your cycle, but you can certainly have a cross-over or find you have winter energy coming through in your spring. This tended to happen to me more if my needs hadn't been met in the menstruation/winter phase.

My psyche wanted me to release and let go of anything that was no longer serving me in winter. I also found an acceptance of the transitions of energy between the phases of each cycle. Naturally we tend to enjoy one or two phases of the cycle more than others. I thought surely everyone loves the spring and summer phases of the cycle the most, right? I found on discussion with others that this is not true. Many women prefer the autumn/winter phases. Through the process, I was able to discover the gifts at each stage. I grew to love my autumn and winter phases too. I could also see how in autumn (which can be a tough phase of the cycle with many negative connotations), I could reframe my understanding to see it as a gift for us, showing us internally what is not working in our lives, or asking us to make changes for more ease in this phase.

I began to plan and utilise my energy to fit in with the changes of my cycle. It was true that I loved taking my boys somewhere in the summer/ovulation phase as I had more energy. If I could plan rest time, it would always be in the menstruation/winter phase.

Think of some of your creative ideas or projects that you could fit into the hormonal shifts of your menstrual cycle. I discussed writing a book into the phases above.

Let's take another example of creating a film. In spring, the pre-ovulation phase, you may start having ideas for your film. This is the time to start planning what you might do, perhaps mind mapping or just journaling. It could feel exciting, and the seeds of your creativity are planted. It is not the phase to broadcast your film to the world.

In the summer ovulation phase, you have high energy and it would be a great time to start filming your scenes. You can start putting your ideas and plans into action. You can nurture your ideas and help them grow.

The autumn phase is the perfect time for editing your film, taking an objective view and looking at what isn't working. The inner critic who makes herself known predominantly in this phase fits perfectly, though be careful that you don't let your inner critic take over, especially in the other times of your cycle.

In the winter phase, do nothing! Wisdom and ideas are formulating but may not manifest yet.

When you start practising and charting the energies of your cycle, it can be a revelation to go deeper into yourself to see where you need to increase self-care or where you haven't addressed emotions or past issues or are not following your inner intuitive guidance.

Over time, as I tracked my own cycle and continued treatments of womb massage with Leora, it has been like peeling back the layers of an onion, parts of my past seeping out in sessions that I had no idea I was holding on to. I revisited unhealed memories, where I had built barriers to protect myself from feeling pain or rejection, as most of us have done, particularly from childhood. All this serves as a disconnection from ourselves. It was a revelation to me, the insights that came forth in our sessions. We will all have had some issues we have pushed into our shadow; it was through this work that I was able to access what I hadn't even realised was there and could begin to empower myself. The more the months passed as I was tracking my cycle, the more I could spot patterns and transitions in my energy and emotions on similar days of every cycle. I was accessing my wisdom and connection to my body. Like a mindfulness practice, I became less frustrated by the shifts of emotions. I was learning to sit with them, seeking their guidance in my life and what that meant for me. I could also see where if I didn't eat or sleep well or had had more stress than usual in a cycle I would be more fatigued or have more symptoms at menstruation. (In the year post the birth of my second child I had symptoms continuously through the cycle.)

I allowed whatever was there to be there, not trying to change it or fight it. If I felt frustrated or angry in the post-ovulation phase of my cycle, I could just question, what was it I needed? Or what did I want to release? It is the acceptance of it all that creates peace and inner happiness and, of course, not comparing your experience to others. Menstrual cycle awareness is also an amazing mindful practice in this regard. I began to welcome the full range of my experiences and emotions, including any rage that might appear. We are not supposed to be stuck; emotions are energy in motion. It is healthy to allow our emotions to be felt. I was observing them come and go and offering the tools of self-care when I needed them. It is a strength, not a weakness, to feel all of your emotions, and it can be tiring if you are constantly hiding from the more difficult ones.

I began listening to what my body needed to balance itself out in each phase of my cycle. If I gave myself what I needed, I could give of myself and help others with more ease; this is the same for us all.

When I looked at where I was in my cycle compared to the moon in its cycle, I learned that I would bleed with the full moon. I had discovered through my own experience and from the teachings of other wise women that this was a time when the shadow side of ourselves could be illuminated. I was learning what I needed to heal and what my truth was—there was no hiding. It was also a time when I was feeling I needed to share what I was learning with the world. Many women will bleed with the new moon which has a different quality, more in tune with nurturing and mothering. I found when I switched to bleeding with the new moon that it had a slightly easier energy flow for me. But wherever you are in your cycle, and if you are floating in a waxing or waning moon phase, track how you feel and acknowledge any gifts or lessons to learn. To work in more depth with the flow and power of your own cycle, visit melanierossiter.com, where you will find my online course, community and workshops on 'Reclaiming the Cyclical Magic of Your Menstrual Cycle.'

As I was healing myself throughout this time, I was simultaneously noticing big shifts in my clients as well.

It felt like I had had a descent of fear, trauma and pain in the year post birth of my second child and was being rebirthed back to myself with a new understanding that everything that had happened to me had led me here to write this book and share this wisdom obtained from the journey with you now. I highly recommend creating something through trauma and pain, it can be very cathartic.

Pain, in hindsight, was one of my greatest teachers. I had to learn that it was ok to look after myself and put myself first. I had to learn to be ok with not "doing" or being "useful." I had to learn to surrender to what was happening as fighting against it was more difficult. I learnt to let go of any form of trying to control an outcome. I learnt that we are still worthy and important even when we cannot "do" anything. I learned to accept help. But most of all I learned to accept my experience in those moments when I had a flare and to be kinder to myself.

I was having great results using self-care techniques to help ensure a healthier menstrual cycle or ward off endo symptoms; for example, the womb massage I discussed previously, castor oil packs, nutrition and Menstrual Medicine Circles as well as other techniques I will discuss.

You may be wondering what a Menstrual Medicine Circle is?

MENSTRUAL MEDICINE CIRCLE

IT IS A journey into your cycle, a process developed by Alexandra Pope and Sjanie Hugo Wurlitzer, founders of the red school, both facilitators of conscious menstruation. They describe their Medicine Circles on their website, (www.redschool.net) as...

"...designed to help restore your inner ecology as women, the natural energetic, psycho-spiritual 'flow' or order of the menstrual cycle, to create a greater feeling of integration and wholeness. The MMC process taps into this inner ecology, helps you to 'read' the flow of the energy, for example, where it is blocked (i.e., where you are stuck) or bursting its banks (i.e., over-stretching yourself) and initiates repair and restoration of that energetic flow; elicits a deeper insight into yourself and any challenges you are dealing with in your life, including of course any menstrual difficulties. And most importantly, it awakens your inner medicine, an energy, a love that is the beginning of a shift or healing. It can be used as part of a one to one coaching session or working with a group of women."

I always journaled after a Menstrual Medicine Circle with Leora who facilitated my circles, and I documented down any visions, insights, or symbols at each phase of my cycle. As with dreams, there is often a message to decode from our subconscious about what is going on for us at a deeper level. Leora would start by guiding me on a journey, using my imagination to step into the different phases of my cycle. I would be guided with visual, associative and somatic clues.

We would work with what came up for me in each cyclical phase. I found that over each session, the background or setting of each phase remained similar. In my spring, there was often the sun and space around me, in summer/ovulation, it was a similar scene and my boys would usually appear. In autumn/post ovulation, it was a barren landscape, dark but with fire burning throughout the scene. It looked like a frightening scene but, interestingly, I felt in my body the power of it, related to the process of letting go and burning what was no longer necessary. A throne would often appear, representing what I felt symbolised the seat of my inner wisdom.

This part of my cycle in one session appeared as a storm in autumn (post ovulation), so in tune with how I felt in each of the cyclical phases but also with what was happening in my life at the time. For example, before my hysterectomy (see hysterectomy section), the storm appeared. I would often see a visual of a Native American who regularly showed up when I journeyed in the winter phase, he appeared in this vision with us both in a boat riding a storm. He kept saying, "keep going, we've got this." I felt a surge of strength from within my body, so powerful that it brought me to tears. Which logically seemed strange at the time because I could often only connect the scenes' meanings after events had happened or I had integrated the messages. But I could truly feel the power of it coming through my body.

That strength stayed with me before and after my procedure. An inner message that I had the courage and strength for what lay ahead.

In my winter phase, I would often see water and the same Native American guide would appear in my mind. He never showed up in the spring/summer phase until after my hysterectomy. Working with Leora, holding a safe space has always allowed me to safely feel supported, which in turn allows me to feel what is wanting to be felt or acknowledged at the time.

I found that throughout the process of discovering some inner truths, it was often not linear or logical and could not always be rationalised. It could be confusing and messy, but eventually I would sense on the inside a transformation or revealing of wisdom.

Whilst doing these journeys that always felt healing and powerful, I could access my "right brain"; the intuitive and subjective side. It opened up my creativity and the part of me that was much stronger earlier on in life, as it is for many of us before other things in life take over. I realised how important it was to reignite my creativity in the way I wanted to. And it was interesting to note that whilst having symptoms in this area, my creativity in life had also become blocked. More on this later.

We also occasionally did EFT (Emotional Freedom Techniques) to release and support the emotions that the womb massage or Menstrual Medicine Circles brought up (see EFT chapter).

Questions to ask yourself for your cycle journal at the end of this book, and what you may need to release:

- Are you speaking your truth?

- Are you people pleasing?

- Are you addressing challenges in your life?

- Are you stuck in some way?

- Is your creativity blocked?

- Do you have unfulfilled dreams?

- Are you feeling disconnected from your body? Do you hear the messages it is giving you? How do you respond?

We can also see the energies or archetypes of the inner life of women in our life stages, known as the Maiden (youth), Mother (obvious!), Enchantress (wild woman) and Crone (wise woman). It doesn't matter which phase of life you are in. Most of us know these archetypes and as with following our menstrual cycle, they can cross over, and we know all three whatever our current age. I do feel each archetype is stronger when we are in that life phase so I am sure I will discover more about the Enchantress and Crone when immersed in these life phases. For more information on the archetypes, you can read Miranda Gray's *Red Moon*.

I will be focusing on my inner interpretation of the Maiden, Mother, Enchantress and Crone; and how I feel these archetypes have played out in me through different life stages and within the menstrual cycle. I am not yet a Crone by life stage; I am entering the Enchantress stage, but we will know these archetypes within us as they play out in the phases of the menstrual cycle, too. Our wisdom with the Crone archetype strengthens as we age. You may have your own unique understanding of how these archetypal traits play out within you.

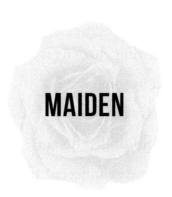

MAIDEN

IN OUR LIFE stage, the Maiden archetype is the time when a woman is in her youth, with more of a focus on the self and self-development. We may be more authentic as the expectations and conditioning of our society haven't yet weighed us down. It can be a time of naivety, innocence, intrigue, curiosity, impatience and taking risks. Think of fairy tales where young women or girls end up in trouble because they haven't used or understood their powers of discernment or haven't trusted their intuition. In life, it is an experimental time. Maidens are developing their senses and wisdom and are learning to trust their gut feelings around people and decisions. I played with all sorts of dangers in this phase of my life. I travelled independently many times and probably put myself in precarious circumstances regularly. I was lucky most of the time, but not always. Upon reflection, I was meeting many people and without thinking about it would go out with them to various places. I would never tell anyone where I was going, so if something had happened, nobody would have known. I was a wild child for sure. I couldn't be told. I liked to find things out for myself and sometimes the hard way, but this phase asks that we experiment but keep our instincts strong. I think that independence was a very important part of building wisdom. If I had been dependent on others too much, I may not have developed a strong inner compass, and this is the same for us all. We live and learn. I would also like you to think about any subliminal messages you may have received in fairy tales surrounding women or girls that may be patriarchal. Love that wild woman within.

In our menstrual cycle, the Maiden links to our pre-ovulation phase with more of a focus on the outside world and our minds, rather than intuition and our inner world.

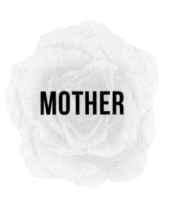

MOTHER

THIS IS THE phase of life I am currently in. It is beautiful and challenging all at the same time. The Mother phase does not mean solely giving birth to children. For women who decide they do not want children, this phase can play out by nurturing a career or business or whatever path chosen. The energies of nurturing and compassion can be strong whatever you are doing in the Mother phase. We must learn to give of ourselves whilst nourishing ourselves too. We cannot give if we are empty ourselves and, if we do, we are likely to be resentful. We can also be Mothers in the wider community in some way. This phase can be difficult as it often involves a lot of juggling. We may have children and older parents to care for, or a busy career and other responsibilities that play out heavily in this phase of our lives, creating disharmony. If you have children, it can sometimes be a difficult transition with the loss of freedom. The focus shifts from the self, but on the other hand is full of love and joy and can be such a positive and beautiful shift. It is always important to honour all emotions that arise in the Mother phase. It can also be a distressing time for women who want children but haven't been able to conceive. We are honing our intuitions and integrating lessons we have learned in the Maiden archetypal phase of our lives. We also do not always get the rest that we need. Make sure you reach out to others, increase your self-care and change what you can so that this archetypal energy can flow with more ease. Learning acceptance and patience has also helped me.

In the menstrual cycle the Mother phase links to ovulation and abundance.

ENCHANTRESS

THIS IS THE phase of perimenopause and transition and the one that is often dreaded, also relating to PMT (pre-menstrual tension). I like some aspects of the "wild woman" in my own life; there is the potential to sift out what isn't working, and to find the truth of our feelings. We can be more forceful in our needs and setting boundaries. The Enchantress is about reflecting and integrating our experiences. It can be challenging, as it relates to the darker and shadowy aspects of our psyches. This archetype aids in our healing as we have to look into our drives and more uncomfortable feelings and integrate them. We can often be unconscious, as I have discovered in my own healing and through working with others. This is where a large part of the difficulty in this phase stems from. We may not understand why we are feeling or behaving the way we are, and our busy lives may not support the time we need to go into the truth around what is asking to be acknowledged and reflected upon. Acceptance is also key, and healing, as I have discovered personally, takes time. I like its unpredictability and rawness. There is no playing the 'good girl' here. Self-care and learning to support ourselves as well as seeking outside support can help this phase.

In the menstrual cycle, the "wild woman" phase relates to post-ovulation and truth-seeking.

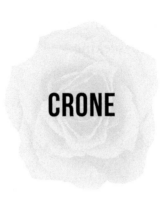

CRONE

CRONE, LIKE THE word "witch," can sometimes conjure up negative connotations of an old cackling woman. Before patriarchy, the word had positive connotations. The archetypal Crone is incredibly wise, and this phase usually comes around our menopause and beyond. Wise women in some cultures are not always respected or accepted for standing in their power. The Crone has strong intuitive and heightened senses. She is wise about the ways of the world and no longer wants to do things that she is not passionate about. She may be far more discerning on how she plans her time, the same when menopausal or post menopause. 'Don't sweat the small stuff' springs to mind when thinking about the Crone. She is also possibly interested in helping with worldly affairs rather than issues closer to home. She may be more interested in creating a legacy, a way to leave the world in a better place for the younger generation. She is likely to know what she wants and be firm with boundaries and her time. Her connection to the earth may be strong and she may have a love of gardening. She will not suffer fools gladly. The Crone knows the dark and the shadows and how to transmute or harness them.

In the menstrual cycle the Crone links to menstruation, a time of stillness and insights.

To give you an idea of how the Maiden, Mother and Crone might play out in a scene…

A girl, let's call her Ruby, meets a boy, let's call him John, and they meet at Ruby's parents' house. John is very polite, almost overly polite, and keeps hold of Ruby's hand. Ruby is smitten, she cannot see what Mother, let's call her Muriel, sees. Muriel senses something is not right with John, she feels he is putting on a front and is picking up on something unsaid. Grandma (Crone) has arrived. Immediately she sees John has a wad of cash in his pocket and knows that there is something going on. John is young, and the amount of money in his pocket is unusual. Grandma straight out asks John where the money is from. Ruby is embarrassed and gets frustrated and angry. How could her grandma be so rude? Her grandma tells her not to argue, grandma knows too much from her experience and her knowing is so strong that she doesn't question it. Muriel gives her mother an enquiring look but is unsure who to stand up for. Her daughter has just been shouted at and her mum has been daring and a little rude in her eyes too. Surely it is none of their business?

John meanwhile is blushing purple and stumbling on his words. He manages to create a story that the money is his mum's that she has given to him to pay for a holiday. Ruby gives a look of "see, you are so rude to ask." She thoroughly believes him through her rose tinted, loved-up glasses. Mother is wanting to be on her daughter's side but knows her mum is probably right. Grandma is still staring intently at John. John makes his excuses and leaves. Outside is a police car waiting for John. He has been dealing in drugs with a friend. Ruby is in tears. Mother is in shock, and grandma holds Ruby, but with a glare, says, "you must get in touch with your intuition."

Ok, this story will not win The Booker Prize, but you catch the drift.

We could make up lots of scenarios around the different archetypes but ultimately in the Maiden life phase we will become discerning and learn from our experiences. We will hopefully begin to listen to our intuition. A Maiden must try to dig for her truth and not get carried away or hold on to the stories the mind creates in relation to her emotions, losing her inner senses. The Crone has a knowing sense; she has developed her wits and trusts herself. Women have this powerful intuitive sense. Let us not lose it, let us hone it.

A vast number of women around the world are beginning to reclaim feminine wisdom. There has been such a disconnection from our femininity and the wisdom inherent in our bodies that many women are suffering or feeling confused and alone with their menstrual pain or disease. Uncertain of the causes if not inherited or passed on down the ancestral line. Many women are not tapped in to the power and inner medicine of their own pelvic bowls. I certainly wasn't.

What makes some countries more prevalent with female conditions such as endo, fibroids, PCOS and so on than others?

Is it the way we live our lives? Our eating habits? Our culture? Our environment? Genetics? Disconnection from our bodies' cyclical wisdom or a true connection to each other? Spiritual disconnection? Or disconnection with ourselves as a part of nature rather than separate from it?

I feel it is a combination of all of these factors.

The shifts in our psyche and bodies through our menstrual cycle and particularly through our rites of passage, such as menarche, motherhood and menopause, often leave women confused and suffering. We have no anchor for these emotional or archetypal shifts when we are not conscious of why they are occurring or how we can work with them. We often relate it to something happening in our external world or life rather than our inner one. Except our inner world affects the perception of our outer world.

Living in a world dominated by and set up for masculine/ yang and linear energy leaves women regularly feeling depleted.

Ever wonder why the men in your life seem to be able to keep going in such a linear fashion whilst you feel somehow inadequate that you cannot follow suit? Ending up feeling like you are on a hormonal rollercoaster and being labelled "crazy woman" when you lose it because you cannot fit into that model?

We think of our reproductive organs as just physical parts that create babies without understanding our female energy system held within our bodies. Our hormones are powerful messengers and when they are imbalanced, it will impact your life in very noticeable ways. Those of you who have experienced any of the energy therapies out there will know how you can shift your emotions and energy through using these therapies and managing and protecting your energy through creating boundaries when you need to. We must also learn to accept where we are in our cycle without trying to change it, which will regularly result in frustration. It's an ongoing challenge.

If we included ceremony, celebration or ritual for a woman at menarche (her first period), this could be good for all women, and I feel strongly that if I had the knowledge and connection to my body then that I do now, I would have loved and honoured my body more. I would have also changed the way I dealt with or understood triggers for endo or cyclical pain. Now more than ever is the best time for mother and daughter to come together and celebrate the daughter's entry into womanhood. Acknowledging the potential for creativity and birthing new life, whether it be a child or a creative project. Menarche is a woman's rite of passage.

Mothers can pass their wisdom on, but herein lies a challenge. If the mother has not had her menarche honoured or celebrated, or she has not been educated about the cyclic wisdom of her cycle, she may not have had any experience of it to pass on or understand the power of it in all aspects of her life. Especially when our culture works against the cyclical energy transitions of women and many have pain, wishing their cycle away. This is understandable. But we can celebrate and honour a woman's menarche at any stage in her life to help create a better relationship to her cycle.

Ritual or celebration could involve just the mother and daughter or if your mother is no longer with you, choose a female close to you. It could also involve family and friends, depending on your preference.

A special gift could be brought for the daughter as a recognition, something like a menstrual cycle tracking diary or journal which could be a great way for her to connect to the different emotions and wisdom she gains as she experiences her cycle. (See the introductory tracking journal at the end of this book.)

If there is pain, this can be tracked, too: Which days? How is her diet? Is there anything emotional occurring in her life alongside the pain? A moon or precious stone ring would also be a nice idea, or a moonstone (related to the feminine) bracelet. Plan your celebration together as mother and daughter, you could decorate with red to represent the bleed. Women can share their experiences, the negative and positive.

The daughter could be presented with a book suggesting advice or guidance to help her navigate through this transition. Imagine how different some of our experiences would be if your first period was celebrated? Would this have affected how you felt about the experience and being female?

Most of us will be given a tampon and a pat on the back, or in some cultures, women have truly been shamed with the idea that periods are dirty. Let us not forget women who cannot afford menstrual products and the issues this brings. We have more of a voice in the West than some other cultures around the world and we must raise our voices for those who really feel they can't.

There are charities that can help women in this position. We also have menstrual products taxed—yep! Nature has a tax on it.

There is also a debate about dioxins produced from bleach used in some menstrual products. As an endo sufferer, I stopped using them, as dioxins can have an adverse effect on the hormonal system and have been linked to endo. Mooncups are becoming more popular and are easier on the environment too. You can buy them in different sizes but keep them clean and sterile to avoid spreading bacteria.

I now always question what I put in and on my body.

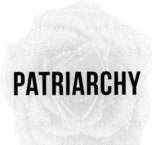

PATRIARCHY

When I discuss patriarchy, I am referring to a large portion of history, and the present to an extent, in which a group of powerful and influential men held authority and created a social system. It held both positive and negative outcomes. Cultures progressed in a linear fashion whereby much of the cyclical wisdom of women and connection to nature was lost, suppressed or rejected, intentionally or otherwise. The notion of 'doing' and a more logical and rational approach to life were encouraged. This is not an argument about genders; this is about bringing the balance of the feminine and masculine back in us all, and praising both. It is about remembering that both are just as important. When I say patriarchy I am referring to it in a sense that it is a system that spread out across most of the world. Of course, there was a dark side to this way of operating, too.

I tell my story because I feel that many women are disconnected from their bodies and cyclical nature and this can cause issues as seen in myself. I could see how many women in my life couldn't get their needs met or had suffered various traumas from their pasts and were suffering menstrual pain. I can only speculate from what I have experienced personally.

Many of us are unable to take time out and most mums no longer live in large families and communities where there is support and help bringing up children. This is a real problem, worse for single parents whether male or female. I have been lucky to have some great mum friends and groups which makes a huge difference to the joy you experience with young kids and the support we all provide for each other. Without this it can be a different experience. Postnatal depression is common, and birth is another area where women can feel disempowered and disconnected.

I still remember thinking to myself when young, if I could be more like a man or please men, I would have more fun, power, and could be successful in the world, because that is what I could see happening around me at that time. I was thinking about how best to fit into a still predominantly patriarchal world to survive and thrive, looking to men for how to succeed and as the more influential of the sexes from my younger vantage point. I hadn't yet realised that masculine energy is generally more linear, outwardly focused and less fluctuating, their hormonal systems wired differently. I was wrong in my thinking, but I didn't question it until later in life. As women, if we try to follow this system, there is a chance that we can quickly become depleted, especially if we are already struggling with hormonal imbalances. I also wasn't taught about the power and cyclical gifts of being female. We can lead in a cyclical feminine way which works best for our bodies and their changing needs but a society that is set up for constant striving and "doing" and fits more naturally into the masculine/yang energy system makes it very difficult. We receive a lot of our wisdom and insights in the second half of our cycle. We can be just as "productive" but in a way that our bodies work with us to be. Many women are learning to lead in this way; if you are self-employed, it is easier. Unless you have a boss that allows flexible ways of working. The challenge remains. If you are a stay-at-home mum, receiving support will hugely help too. But you can start to make small changes or self-care practices to fit into your changing needs.

From an early age, I was curious about the world and felt ambitious. I was never very good at being told what to do or how I should live my life, especially to fit into a role. I believe men and women are suffering from trying to fit into defined gender "roles."

Many men feel they cannot express their feelings for fear of judgement with a perception that it is not a "male" thing to do. Unfortunately, male suicide rates are far too high.

This was in part my journey into how I could love my feminine body and what the truth was from my inner feminine nature, especially as endometriosis and postnatal trauma had caused so much disruption and instigated so many questions.

The revealing wisdom and gifts of feminine mystery through the work I was doing began to make me frustrated at the loss of understanding in our culture of feminine beauty and wisdom, and I am not talking about the bombardment of the perfect female body from the media that serves women to become further disconnected from themselves and their inherent inner wisdom, in turn making women dislike their bodies. Men are struggling with this too. We are hearing more cases of male anorexia or men down at the gym every day, striving for the "perfect" body.

I wanted to know why as women we often do not give our bodies what they desire or need and what the effect of this is from a holistic perspective. What roles are we living out and why? How is our society and patriarchy affecting a woman's body to this day? Where is the support? It's time to break the silence.

We can refer to history to see how women have been portrayed. I like to go by my own experiences to gain insights and wisdom. But our cultures are still affected by the stories or the historical religious backgrounds we grew up in. There was a great programme that came out just before I started writing this book called, *Jesus' Female Disciples: The New Evidence*, (created by Minerva Media in association with Jerusalem Productions for Channel 4 which was broadcast on the 8th of April 2018).

Academics Helen Bond and Joan Taylor felt that the female disciples of Christianity had slowly been removed from the picture of the faith and erased from historical references. They proceeded to set out on a journey to try and unearth this truth. Ancient historic references show how women were perhaps far more prominent in early Christianity than we have been led to believe. The documentary highlighted that it may well have been women who helped finance the movement of early Christianity and were necessary to its growth, but many will not have heard about that.

We can see how women may have been losing status and power through powerful male figureheads of that time and many history books were written by men. This is one example. We must always question what we are presented with and the underlying messages we receive. We must also question our deeply held beliefs whilst looking at how we operate in the world before we can transform or change our stories.

What are our feminine or masculine truths? And what is the balance in ourselves without the interplay of our culture or conditioning in society? What is feminine and masculine if both have been distorted? Are they solely constructs?

As women, the majority of us may have lost touch with feminine practices and truths. We also have a history of witch hunts, women set against each other for survival, or burned for their knowledge of herbs or because they were midwives. Is this still in the feminine consciousness and psyche somehow?

I reclaimed the word 'witch' for myself, uncovering how patriarchy burned women alive because they used their natural feminine gifts in the world, shaming and driving women underground. Lisa Lister's book *Witch* is a fantastic read regarding reclaiming the word and she has a lot to say about patriarchy.

We can also question the language that we use, and the words that carry meaning. A recent post on Facebook that went viral by Fleasay Malay, a spoken word artist and poet, called "Witches" highlights this perfectly. She is part of the wave of women beginning to speak out at the truth behind the word, and questioning the shame held by women surrounding speaking out about many things, particularly with regard to their sexuality. If we do not acknowledge the roots of our shame, we can become disempowered.

The word witch to me used to conjure up images of an old woman cackling on a broomstick; in nursery rhymes, she is to be feared and is often portrayed as evil, a parody. In the past, I would never have liked to call myself a witch. Hence the need to question our language and its connotations. Now I would tattoo it on my forehead: Witch = woman in her power and sharing her voice and gifts. Not afraid to say no or speak her truth—I am a witch in this regard, pleased to meet you.

You will also often hear people say, "that took balls," never "ovaries"! There is so much in our language that we do not question.

The reason this word began to interest me was because I would have been burned for the work I do today under the rules for burning "witches," as so many of us would have been. There is still a lot of fear around the word based on its history, and we are meant to be afraid of its connotations. If they wanted to name certain women "witches" and associate the word with negative connotations, we can reclaim it as a positive word for women who were burned unjustly. But ultimately, it's a word. It's the meaning, the historical undertones, of what patriarchy wanted it to represent and the fear they wanted it to produce which makes me want to reclaim it for women who were burned for their work in the world. Whether it was fear from a misunderstanding of the source of a women's power in those days, or an intentional way to subjugate women.

And so, from an early age I had no initiation and celebration into the power and beauty of the female body. The qualities of receiving, intuition, creativity, cycles, sensuality and rhythm. My first period was not celebrated, and there was no initiation into the power and wisdom held in my menstrual cycle; so few of us know this. I now have a recognition of the force of nature and mystery inherent in women's bodies. I have this whilst living with endo and a history of being frustrated by having to have a period. We just haven't been taught how it can affect our creativity and be a guide to reducing stress and showing us what needs addressing in ourselves. We are collectively suffering through our wombs, and they may be trying to tell us something about the way many of us are living. You could say the cyclical element of this book is "ode to my womb" and the lessons I learned, as you are about to find out why I decided to have a hysterectomy.

When I delved deeper into my cycle, I felt robbed of knowledge that could have helped me in every area of my life to realise that it was normal to not want to be on the go all the time, to accept the beauty of receiving rather than striving continuously. The need for self-care and the discomfort of going against our bodies' natural rhythms. This only causes stress, and stress wreaks havoc on our hormones and reproductive system. Too much cortisol too often affects hormonal balance and the digestive and immune system. Progesterone is especially affected by the adrenal glands pumping out cortisol. Low levels can cause headaches, low libido, hot flashes, anxiety and depression. This in turn affects our moods and fertility if trying to conceive. If you have endo, I have tracked closely enough to see a very clear correlation to stress and an endo flare, also affected by the hormonal imbalance caused by stress. By using the self-care practices in this book, you can begin to work with any stressful situations in a different way. I have found it imperative. Meditation and mindfulness are especially effective.

I am so grateful to have eventually come to this knowledge, and for myself and many others, our wish is for younger women to be more educated in how to acknowledge and look after the shifting energies and hormonal changes inherent in the menstrual cycle, flowing with rather than against it and harnessing its power in our lives. We need menstrual education is schools so women have more understanding of their changing hormonal experiences and needs. And of course so that girls are aware of when something is not right and they may be experiencing a menstrual condition or disease. We need to start respecting and connecting to the power of the female body because it has been silenced for too long. We also need to demand better research into conditions such as endometriosis and women need to be respected for their decisions with regard to their health.

Menstrual cycle awareness has truly helped me to surrender to the ebb and flow of life. If anything, this has been the biggest message. Allow the shifts in the psyche and body to move through you and the insights to emerge. It is easier to feel into what you want to express in the world, or what is best for you, if you can allow the space for it to come in. The more we are trying to control our lives, the harder we can make it for ourselves. What if what we are striving for is not actually what is best for us? Have you ever worked hard for something only to find out it is not what you wanted after all?

I know I have. Allow time and space for your gifts to emerge and listen to your passions.

SO, WHAT ABOUT MEN?

FOR MEN, THERE was an article in *Kindred Spirit* by author and coach Michael Boyle who discusses an initiation for men, the "Mankind Project."

He highlights that menarche is a natural initiation for womanhood but argues the case that men have no clear entry to manhood. He states in the article that:

"Manhood is a social construct and therefore needs to be accomplished and externally conferred by 'others' who are regarded as judges or authorities. Manhood was, and is, something that always has to be proven and therefore has always been difficult to feel secure about. So, it is inevitably tinged with ego, over-confidence and often a tendency towards risk."

He discusses tribes with male tribal elders who emphasise the importance of an initiation for men. He also refers to the instinct in males to seek initiation and how this unmet need can play out in adulthood and how this loss has played out in men throughout most of the world. He discusses the issues of mental health in men who are struggling with anxiety and depression. I am obviously not male so cannot comment from experience, but I can certainly see his argument.

We are all victim to our cultures and conditioning, but we can dig deep and question and come to spiritual and emotional recognition of what we are losing out on and how we can rekindle our losses.

Interestingly, he also discusses how in this project men can drop their roles and become vulnerable, also what we as women do in circle. I have found the more vulnerable and honest we are, the more others will open up to us in true connection. This is the same for us all.

HYSTERECTOMY – HUH?

MY STORY DID not end in the way a fairy tale would. I imagine as you are reading this book, you would find it difficult to understand why I decided to have a hysterectomy. But despite having amazing results with everything I was doing, I had a deep sense of something needing or wanting to happen, and even I was surprised by it. It was not the way I felt it would lead when journeying with the healing and cyclic wisdom, especially after much joy and success with it. I am so grateful to have made the discoveries.

If I had been in the right frame of mind whilst waiting for the operation with the retained placenta, I may have chosen to have a hysterectomy then. Had I known the anxiety and months of pain that would follow, as well as the loss of joy experienced with my newborn until I then had to have another surgery for the mess it had left behind, I may have chosen differently. I was told I might lose my womb, but I do not remember ever being given the option. I also would not have experienced the utter blessing and gifts that followed, the mini miracles, and synchronicities. I would not have experienced any of the joy of reconnection to myself and to the beautiful, amazing women I met on the way. I would not have the understanding or respect of a woman's body that I do now and I would not be able to work to the spiritual and emotional depth I am able to work with other women. I believe everything happened exactly as it was meant to.

That is why after doing much journeying and healing with my cycle and wise sisters, I had the insight through doing the inner work with myself that it was still to be a part of my unfolding story to have this operation. I had understood through womb work what I needed to heal and learn. It had returned me to the feminine mysteries and the cyclical wisdom and power within. I had started to have a return of some symptoms around my right ovary after over a year. I felt I had come to a crossroads. I had kept my surgeon, but I knew it would not be long before I would have to let him go as he could not keep me on his system forever. I had to make my decision.

Was I going to let him investigate what had really happened inside after the birth of my second child? Was there anything else I still needed resolving? I knew I had my symptoms under control and I had loved so much tracking my cycle and learning from it, but I was getting a deep inner call that this was to be the step I should take. I couldn't even understand this myself. I had stopped many of my symptoms. I had been blessed in the discoveries I made. Why was I feeling this way? Where was this feeling coming from? I realised I wanted him to clear any remnants of anything left behind, including the scar tissue in my womb, and I felt I did not want my womb to be scraped or burned again. I felt a lot of damage had already been done and I was tired of it. I wanted to release my womb in a way that would release the trauma that it had been through and to clear up the mess that I felt was left inside from the experience. I had come to peace with what happened, and with my endo, so I felt I was able to do this in a way that would work for me. I had gone from hating to loving my womb and all it represented. It had helped me to rediscover a deep respect for the feminine.

I also found out afterwards that my surgeon was going fully private. Despite having the initial consultation with him privately, I was referred through the NHS for surgery, again, another synchronicity in the timing. It is a huge shame that we are losing another skilled endo surgeon to private healthcare that many will not be able to afford.

To say I didn't have worries and fears though is a lie. It's major surgery. My mind kept repeating, what if something happens? What if you are left worse off? What if you lose this powerful connection you have made? What about all the women I had helped? What would they think?

There came the shame, bubbling up, the worries about how it would be perceived, of being judged, by others and myself, the exact thing I wanted women to stop doing to each other. Judgement is often related to something we need to look at in ourselves. It's healthier to be kinder about our predicaments and decisions, whether they turn out for the best or not.

Many women who have had hysterectomies have said it was a positive experience for them. I had always been able to see different points of view, but it's important not to judge another woman's decision on what to do with her body. Some women regret it and can experience negative outcomes, others feel much better. There might not be a choice to make, in some cases. It is, however, for many women a tough decision to make. Especially for women that haven't been able to have children. Remember that it is a decision that must be made by us and that women can have unnecessary hysterectomies that they have been told they should have, though they may have had other options, whether medical or holistic. You may want some time to discover alternate routes, unless, of course, it's a medical emergency and has to be removed for your safety. I found it far more emotional having grown to love my womb and the menstrual cycle than I would have done beforehand. I would have been happy to have one before I discovered the gift it was. But I was also very grateful and it felt like the right time to let go.

The shame I felt had to be released. What would I say to a client? I would do exactly as Leora had done for me. Held space for women on their journey. Now I needed to do the same for myself.

I, of course, did take time to explore it and check in with myself to see why I was feeling this way after such an incredibly special year.

I felt a desire to meet with Andrea Clarke. She had been a mentor with Leora on my womb massage training course. She is also one of the few (at the time of writing) currently in the UK who is trained by Tami Lynn Kent who developed Holistic Pelvic Care.

Tami is also the author of *Wild Feminine* and a female physiotherapist, energy worker and teacher, having designed her own method of working through her experiences treating women with pelvic and gynaecological conditions. Through working with many women, originally on the physical mechanics of the pelvis, she began to witness and acknowledge the emotional pain and the shame held by women in this area. Her experiences of connecting with women showed her that there were more than physical issues at play. She has presented her experiences and insights in a Ted talk.

I have already discussed how my own shame held in the pelvic bowl would arise through womb work and where I have seen this with the women I work with. This sense of shame allowed me to see where I had disconnected from my body and where other women were disconnecting from theirs. Women can feel shame around many things. A common example is a woman who has been sexually abused, she hasn't felt safe to share her experience because she wonders if she brought it on herself by wearing a short skirt or being too drunk, or because she was flirting too much. She worries about how she will be perceived or judged, and if she will be believed, she feels disempowered. Feeling a sense that it is not safe to share her experiences. Resulting in inner turmoil.

See if you can pinpoint any areas of your life where you don't feel comfortable sharing because it doesn't feel safe. The more we open up about where we are feeling shame, the easier it will be to understand that we are often just victims of trauma or that we have past issues that we haven't healed or accepted with love. It really is a collective issue for women. I have also seen women feel guilty about expressing boredom around the more mundane parts of motherhood, myself included, or women who are trying to conceive feeling as if there must be something wrong with them if it hasn't happened, feeling they can't talk about it to others. This feeling of not being able to share and the guilt of unaccepted feelings turns inwards, as I said in the beginning, to manifest as unwarranted shame. It's worth being aware of any labels put upon women such as 'slut' or the 'virgin, good girl' this adds to disempowerment. Own your sexuality.

The treatment I experienced from Andrea was powerful, and as we were talking, I remember her saying to me, "it's amazing what happens when we give our power away."

In this moment it hit home again. It can be applied to so many situations—having sex when you don't feel like it, or not trusting your own wisdom or intuition. Believing another's guidance for you over your own and later finding out that your hunches were right, creating frustration with yourself for not trusting or acting upon your own inner knowing.

Where in your life do you give your power away? Especially with regards to seeking validation from others when you already know your answers?

It was this that helped clarify my decision the most, it was from within me that I received the instinctual message to do this, and it was intuitively too strong to ignore. I could not give my power away worrying about how it would be received by others and I needed to stop second guessing myself. With all that had happened over the year, I knew I had to trust this. It sounds strange but even if things did go wrong, I still knew it would be something I had felt I needed to do, like a sense of completion of the trauma that occurred. I knew I would still be prone to endo or possibly not have every part removed, especially in the thoracic area, but I knew that I was way more empowered to work with it and had a full action plan and toolkit.

I booked the surgery.

One thing I was certain about was that I had learnt the power and magic in ritual and sacred ceremony. I was going to do a ritual to release my womb before the surgery and my beautiful guide Leora would facilitate it for me. We did the stunning practice of womb massage where Leora would guide me on a meditative journey, and what came into my mind, yet again, was my Native American. He was riding a dolphin and I was given the message to follow the dolphins. I remember laughing with Leora afterwards thinking, where was I going to see a dolphin?

I am laughing right now at how ridiculous this sentence might come across to you. Just think of dreams but being in the state where you are conscious of what is happening. Receiving messages from an altered state of consciousness and accessing our subconscious for what we have repressed, sleep and dreaming are said to be an altered state of consciousness. I was always able to come out of the journey whenever I wanted.

I had brought a rose quartz crystal with me and Leora had placed it on my chest. I had a visual of the dolphin playing with the crystal and received the message to follow my heart. It was a beautiful ceremony, and I always felt an energetic shift after our work. I expressed gratitude to my womb for bringing me my beautiful children and all the wisdom it took me a long time to realise it held.

I knew I would keep that crystal with me especially through surgery.

The next day, I received a postcard from my parents who had been travelling around Australia. In it they said they had seen some beautiful dolphins swimming by their boat. I told Leora who then told me that her first client had had a dolphin tattoo. I then picked my *Osho Zen Tarot* card for the day, "harmony" with a picture of dolphins swimming towards a heart, and I had been told to follow my heart. That night, my husband put the television on and, you guessed it, dolphins.

I received a letter from the hospital that stated I would be staying in for one night after the procedure, but it was supposed to be three nights, so this was my first setback. I had organised to stay in Birmingham the night before the surgery and I had to take bowel prep to cleanse the bowel as he would be working around it. My husband showed up that night after work and dropping the kids at Granny's house and then taken the two and a half hour drive to be with me. All was going fine until just past midnight when I was sick from the prep.

Game over, surgery cancelled. I smiled because life had other plans. I wasn't thrilled with the date I had been given, as it was before Christmas and we were going to be moving to a new house. It would not have been the right time and I felt a little relieved. We would be able to enjoy Christmas with the boys and of course, move to our new house.

I was booked in again at the end of January 2018 on the full blue moon (a rare occurrence when there is more than one full moon in the calendar month). I had heard that a full moon is not great for surgery as there can be an increase in bleeding; just as the tides are moved by a full moon, I believe we are, as our bodies contain water, and my connection to the moon with my cycles had only increased my awareness. I had decided this time that I would stay at home and then we would drive up early in the morning. I had requested a different bowel prep this time, so was hoping I wouldn't get sick again.

Everything was going so smoothly. If anything, it seemed a little odd how good I was feeling, considering it was major surgery. I was ready to go ahead with it and pleased with my decision to stay home and take the prep instead of going up the day before. I had my bag packed and at 3:30 am, we set out on this amazing full moon to hospital. I felt completely calm and surprisingly in good spirits, considering I was going for a major operation to take my womb, which I discovered had been such a source of wisdom and healing, as well as providing me with my two lovely children. I remember arriving early and being so pleased that the organisation and pre-op had gone well. I was sent to my room to be prepped for surgery and was met by a lovely nurse. We were chatting and laughing. I felt fully supported in my journey to get here and had the rose quartz crystal as well as wearing my grandma's opal ring; she had passed away not long before. Unfortunately, the nurse made a comment about how much she liked opal rings, but she then highlighted the superstition that they were supposed to bring bad luck. Not exactly the sort of thing I had wanted to hear before major surgery. It was my grandma's ring and I loved it and was glad it was with me, but what a timely comment!

And so, the morning went on, and on, and suddenly it was 11:00am. I had been in since 6:00am, and it was clear I was not going to be first on the list. A nurse eventually came back and told me that I was in fact last on the list. My heart sank. I know my body and the starvation and bowel prep was beginning to get to me. I was fading, and as the hours slipped by, so did my mood. It was around 3:00pm when a nurse entered and broke the news. The first surgery had taken longer than they expected, and I was taken off the list. My surgeon would not have the theatre time. This time there was no relief. I cried. All that preparation, twice? Cancelled twice? Am I missing something here? I thought. It was not lost on me, and I suddenly began to smile despite my frustration to get here, including the two hour journey, no sleep and no food. I knew, in my heart, that it still wasn't the right time. I did not hold onto the frustration. I let it go and trusted that it just wasn't meant to happen at that time, again!

If I was going to recommend any spiritual practice, it would be the process of letting go and surrendering to what is. As I stated before this can happen when you are bleeding on your period and naturally releasing what hasn't served you in a cycle. If you connect to it, you can truly practice that.

I knew that I was going to have to regain my strength for the next time it would be booked in. I felt I needed to see my wise sister Leora. I needed a womb massage. Was I missing something? Why was I not running for the hills? It was not lost on me, considering the deep work I had been doing.

In meditation after all this happened, I was visualising a lone wolf at the end of my bed, watching me. Not in a frightening way, it was more as a protection or a support. I had to regain myself; the journey wasn't over, and there was still something missing before this surgery was going to happen.

It was great to see Leora. We hugged, and, on the way, I felt like I didn't need to do any "work" with my healing. By this I mean journeying to uncover anything that I hadn't processed in the past. I felt I needed support and, as always, we were on the same page. I didn't need to say anything about this to Leora. Before I opened my mouth, she stated that this was the intention for the session. And so, I had a beautiful treatment where I just felt held and supported.

It would be around four weeks until I was booked in again for surgery. I used that time to regain my strength; this had turned into a particularly lengthy process. A couple of days before the surgery, I wanted to see Leora again, for one last time. I am sure that without the journeying, wisdom, support and lessons I had integrated, this wait period that I had to go through again would have been much more frustrating and worrying. I had acknowledged some inner wisdom and was being given the opportunity to use it.

I had booked in again for the fertility/womb massage with Leora, which had been such a huge part of my healing journey and had become a real passion of mine to give and receive.

Except I felt whilst driving to see her that it was going to turn into a session of EFT (Emotional Freedom Technique). I could feel the emotion rising. I didn't know why at the time, but I knew a hidden and unhealed part of me had something to say. EFT is a powerful therapy that uses the fingers to tap on energy meridians situated on the face and body—acupuncture without needles (I include a section on EFT towards the end). The focus is on releasing energetic emotional imprints held in the body. I was amazed at how effective this treatment was the first time I used it. In sessions, I always felt surprised by what I was holding on to.

When I reached Leora, she had felt the session was to be EFT too, even though I hadn't said anything about it; the universe was beginning to regularly work in mysterious ways to me, and I loved that. I found these sessions the most emotionally painful but very effective. Whilst tapping on an emotion regarding a previous situation, I could literally feel the emotion quietening as I tapped, until it didn't have the same charge.

We would find a situation from my early childhood arise, a belief that had been created that caused a barrier or mistruth to be held, such as "I cannot be loved unless (insert belief)."

As an adult, I could see how these beliefs had set the course for my life; not always in a negative way, sometimes positive, but they had left an imprint. I could now talk to my inner child or journal about the incident and realise that the belief could no longer serve me or have the same hold over how I interacted with the world. Certain situations can provoke outdated responses when we aren't conscious of an unhealed or unprocessed trauma from our past.

It was a potent session, and when I arrived, Leora presented to me a necklace I had brought after my fertility/womb therapy and training. I had taken it to one of her workshops almost a year prior at the start of my healing journey and had left it in the middle of our circle. Often in the red tent or women's circles you may be asked to bring something which represents the feminine.

She had forgotten to ask me if it was mine and I had never asked her for it back. The look we gave each other was again of a deep knowing. It was really time now. It was not a "coincidence," it had to be given to me then, after this last healing session and truly this time before my third attempt at surgery. Not only this, but I had left an aquamarine bracelet with her in our last session that I'd held throughout. It dawned on me that the third time this surgery had been booked was exactly a year since my training with Clare Spink that had been the start of my awakening to the power held in the pelvic bowl. There was so much magic and synchronicity in the lead-up to this surgery. It would be a year I would never forget, a rollercoaster and a catalyst for growth and transformation. The third time the surgery was booked in was truly a completion of a cycle; one year exactly.

There is a lot that we as women have forgotten. I was not leading from my feminine cyclical energy or core as I have highlighted throughout. I was trying to live from a yang/masculine energy all the time, forgetting the gifts and importance of the yin/feminine energy. This is where as women we need to acknowledge and lead from our own sources of wisdom, using our body as a guide. The feminine wants to receive, our bodies need attention and support. I have found, along with many others, that we can be MORE effective in the world and healthier when we work with our natural rhythms and our bodies messages.

And so, I now no longer have my womb. It turned out after seeing my surgeon post-surgery that I had stage four endometriosis on my bladder, womb, pelvic side walls and adhesions in many places. I remember in one of my womb massage sessions saying to Leora that I could see spiders in my mind crawling over my abdomen and pelvis. I associated them with their spider webs, which to me represented the adhesions that I felt were there. As I mentioned in the beginning, I had not had surgery with a specialist endo surgeon the first time. It was my body and intuition's way of telling me what was still inside. I believe the majority of this came around after the operations and I am in no doubt that if I had not been guided to these amazing modalities and wise women at the right time, I probably would have been in pain and would not have enjoyed that second year with all the gifts, spiritual enrichment and personal growth that it brought me.

The ritual and release I had done was also surrounding the trauma that had occurred with my womb, so it had energetically created space. I had trusted the power of intuition and inner knowing. These traits tend to be ridiculed or at least not praised in the way that logic and rationality are. But from a logical perspective I had taken the option to have it with a specialist I trusted. You could argue it was a balanced decision!

Straight after the recovery I felt the call to tell my story. I also felt a powerful desire to be creative again. The ovaries for women are said to be related energetically to creativity and mine had been freed from adhesions. The physical changes had also affected my internal state. This no longer surprised me.

If you are suffering with menstrual pain, I would love you to try as much as you feel you want to from this book to see for yourself if it could support you. I do not believe that because I had a hysterectomy that this is the way forward or route that women with endo or other menstrual conditions should take. It is important to state that a hysterectomy is not a cure for endo. It is also important to have all endometriosis excised at the same time by a skilled surgeon if taking this option. It does not mean that the endo will not grow back.

I had amazing relief with everything I did, and it was a blessing to uncover these therapies. There are many others who do cycle awareness, womb massage, Womb Yoga, Menstrual Medicine Circle, and other healing arts who have drastically reduced or eradicated pain and disease too, and this has not been their ending or call. My story will be as unique as yours. As I stated earlier, I would never judge a woman on any path she would take with her body. These practices could support you with whatever choices you make.

It was also at the time of writing this book that I had the first Menstrual Medicine Circle with Leora after my hysterectomy. This session was very special to me. As I took the journey through my cycle, the same visions appeared at each stage in many ways, but there were differences this time. In the autumn of my cycle, rather than a barren landscape, there were shoots growing out and the messages were clear. It was time to share my voice. The seeds I had planted were beginning to grow. The burning landscape I had seen in the autumn phase of my cycle had disappeared. I could now see a rebirth of plants in the barren landscape. What a metaphor for where I was in my life! I was entering a time of rebirth and new creativity.

This time, my Native American who always popped up in my journeys, was giving me a gift. I had always been a little wary of seeing him at first, but I was clear he needed to be there and that he held a source of power. These subconscious and symbolic messages often hold meaning. He had entered the spring stage of my cycle when usually I saw him in the winter/menstruation stage of my cycle. The message I felt was not to be worried about seeing him throughout my entire cycle. I believe this related to menopause for me.

I would urge all women to work with their cycle and harness their own inner teacher. This was my overall message; to know that all along I have known what is best for me and that we must trust our intuitive knowing and inner wisdom. How often have you wished you had gone with your gut instinct, but you talked yourself out of it?

As I have kept my ovaries, I still feel like I am going through a cyclical process and am very grateful that I had a huge burst of energy and creativity for a good few months afterwards. Interestingly, around half a year later I had a stressful and emotional couple of weeks which then correlated with a return of some thoracic, bladder and abdominal symptoms that I had had in the past. This is likely some endo that wasn't removed in the surgery and some adhesion discomfort or a return of some disease. I realised I was eating many foods that I had cut out previously and had stopped with an anti-inflammatory diet. I also realised, as it was summer, I had been wearing a lot of sun cream, and the chemicals in some brands have been linked to endo as hormone disruptors. I was able to act very quickly to address this (see nutrition section). I realised I had slipped back into a predominantly yang mode, which is easier to do without the cycle to guide and remind you to slow down and receive. I also stopped everything I was doing to take a couple of weeks to rebalance and reduce stress, using the toolkit of techniques in this book to help. I did a Menstrual Medicine Circle whilst having the flare and it was all focused on the autumn/winter part of my cycle. The visual and somatic clues all related to empowerment and bringing light into the dark, representing my need to use what I had learned. I also kept feeling like I was being shown something by my body, which I believe I was. I understood that since I didn't have a womb anymore I couldn't release in the way we do when we bleed so this may have been a reaction as I had been stressed leading up to it. I needed to use EFT or another technique to relieve tension or emotional charge. I also spent a couple of weeks detoxing.

All the tools I used resulted in an almost complete reduction of symptoms. It required me to be patient and to trust my body to rebalance itself. I still have a few in the thoracic area, and I work with adhesions through exercise and castor oil packs. At the time of writing, I am not having discomfort with them, although this may change. It was a reminder of how we can empower ourselves, too. I felt I was being tested to live the methods in this book again. You could say I view myself as a guinea pig for endo and finding other ways to manage symptoms. I didn't see it that way in the year when I was really struggling with pain and not really knowing why or what to do. I feel surgery in my case has benefitted me alongside these practices, although I am hoping to stick with a completely holistic route now as I have more experience and understanding of how to manage it in this way. Know that whatever decision you take with endo, there is hope, and you can empower yourself. I have experienced how effective a combination of holistic therapies, deep self-care and reconnecting with our bodies and their rhythms can be. By tracking my cycle, I have also seen what has happened in my life that has triggered any symptoms to return, and what has been most effective in reducing them. I now focus my work on the importance of what it means to lead from and rediscover our feminine nature. You can download free resources and join my online community based around working with your cyclical nature to drastically enhance your life at melanierossiter.com. The emotional/spiritual link has been the most interesting for me.

For some women, very good excision surgery, or a full holistic programme has eradicated all symptoms of endo and they have not experienced a return. I hope to highlight this the most as often you will not hear from women who are getting on with their lives in most endo groups. It's good to look for the positive stories to know that relief is possible but there needs to be far greater support for anyone who is struggling from the debilitating effects it can have. Others may have had a long break from symptoms but then the disease manifests again, so always look after your body with self-love and care whatever decisions you take. Patience has been a key for me on the holistic path as it's not necessarily a quick fix and my healing was not linear. We are used to being able to do things quickly to create immediate change, but our bodies are not machines. I have loved all of the discoveries.

I am still aware of having all the shifts in my psyche that I had with my menstrual cycle, although they are not following the same pattern and they may become less clear as the archetypal energies merge into each other if I enter early menopause. This is normal, to have different shifts in perimenopause. I track the lunar cycle against my cyclical shifts now to use this as my guide, I know when I am too much in a yang energy because my body warns me.

Having spoken to women who have felt grief that surprised and shocked them after their hysterectomies, I feel even more strongly that our female connection to our cycles and support with feminine therapies and feminine wisdom can help with transition. Many women are disconnected from their bodies or unaware of what is happening with these energetic, hormonal and archetypal shifts. This causes confusion as to why they may be feeling a certain way, often relating it to something outside of themselves rather than what is happening within them. For those who perhaps hadn't wanted a hysterectomy in the first place, the transition may be harder with the loss of a cyclic rhythm and a changing inner landscape. There is a need to ramp up the self-care and support through menopause too.

HYSTERECTOMY RITUAL

THERE ARE MANY ways you could release your womb through a ritual or ceremony process if you know of anyone that has had to have one, or if you find yourself in that position.

I found it so powerful and important to grieve and give gratitude for what it had given me. I know many women will be mixed in how they feel about this surgery; you can do whatever you feel comfortable with. Doing a womb meditation or connection is a powerful start and then setting the intention for release. You can tap on any fear around the surgery, too. You might want to journal your fears and worries and then burn the writing for release or you can ask someone to ceremony with you. You may want to bury something that represents your womb into the earth or offer a letter of gratitude. I had a rose quartz crystal with me throughout for mine and found it powerful to do the womb massage with Leora and journeying into any messages. Just see what comes to you. You could have a few people and create an archway with the woman who is having the surgery coming through to represent transition into the next phase post-surgery. The women creating the archway could offer positive affirmations on the walk through. I imagine many of you might cringe at this, but it can be powerful!

I am so pleased and grateful that I did the ceremony before mine as I found it helped me through the surgery and I released what I needed to. Again, setting the scene with lighting, flowers, oils, artwork or anything that will help create a sacred space adds to the power of the ritual process.

ADDITIONAL HEALING MODALITIES I USED ALONG THE WAY.

HOW I OVERCAME HEALTH ANXIETY.

I HAD SUFFERED from health anxiety in the year after my second son was born because I didn't know what was going on inside my body. I had a good idea, but there was a lot of fear that I may not get better or that it could be more life-threatening. I feel in part that it also had a lot to do with the postnatal hormonal imbalance that was raging inside. The main fear was that something was going to happen to me that would leave my boys without a mum. This is a normal fear that most mums might feel at times, but it had become a problem for me after a traumatic time.

Mostly in Western culture, we often feel we need to control our lives in some way, and so losing a sense of control over my thoughts and what was happening to my body was frightening. The trauma from haemorrhaging had not been processed or healed in me, and that sense of having to keep moving forward to look after my boys was causing an internal struggle and conflict with what my body needed from me.

Often, whether it's conscious or not, there is a part of us that feels that the anxiety is protecting us in some way. This makes sense for my situation because the trauma had caused me to feel unsafe in life. Suddenly the world, in my mind, was not a safe place to inhabit. Irrational thoughts began to spiral as my mind went into overdrive thinking again what other dangers I might encounter that could be life threatening.

Thankfully, all this passed eventually as I learned not to follow the thoughts, but more importantly, the behaviours. For example, googling health symptoms for reassurance. Sure, this may have made me feel better for a short time, but then it becomes a cycle. This applies to any anxiety you may feel in any area of your life, following the anxious thoughts that manifest in behaviours that feel protective but just keep the cycle of anxiety going. If you have anxiety surrounding any area of your life that has become problematic, I suggest you seek professional support from qualified therapists. CBT (cognitive behavioural therapy) is a great start. Reaching out to others is imperative. I hadn't started using many of the methods in this book when I was addressing it but they can support too.

I overcame my anxiety through not following the thoughts and behaviours that continued the cycle. From a holistic perspective, I also used meditation, self-love, and acceptance of what had happened to me. I also worked on healing my gut after a month's worth of antibiotics, and I will explain why this was important later. I also felt that sharing in the women's circles gave me the space to experience being held by other women as I released the emotions surrounding what had happened rather than trying to deal with it all in my head. It was a magical journey in the end. Allowing grief to be felt aids the process. You can use the tools in this book to help.

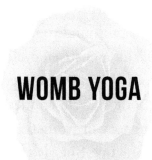

WOMB YOGA

WOMB YOGA WAS created by Uma Dinsmore Tulli, author of *Yoni Shakti*. This form of yoga is entirely grounded in respect and honour for the menstrual cycle, and for all stages of women's life initiations including menarche, pregnancy, postnatal recovery and menopause. Uma highlights…

"Womb Yoga is not really just about postures at all. There are many feminine moves and rhythms in Womb Yoga that respect female bodies—but fundamentally it is a multidimensional yoga practice that also teaches breath awareness, deep relaxation, meditative techniques and consciousness of emotional and psychological experiences related to the menstrual cycle."

The last thing I ever wanted to do was to be active when I had my period, especially with endo. I actually used to wonder how women managed it when it came to exercise at that time of the month. You could end up resentful of your practice if it becomes more like a chore. This happened every time I tried to attempt unsupportive forms of exercise for my cycle.

To honour our cycle through yoga, taking into account the rise and fall in energy is a really nourishing self-care practice. The worst thing you can do is push yourself at times when your body is saying no.

Womb Yoga is not a form of exercise, it is a holistic self-care practice that utilises profound yoga practices to nourish and support every phase of the menstrual cycle.

Uma has developed Womb Yoga practice and is a source of wisdom for women's bodies, cycle connection and menopause. She has explored the history of women in yoga and the politics of contemporary yoga practice. She also discusses the manifestations of Shakti in our lives, Shakti being referred to as life force.

Whilst doing all of my womb work, I often began to notice I would get tingles rising up my spine from the base whenever I felt I or someone else was discussing a truth. It was new for me to connect to this, but through my own deepening experience, I began to obtain clearer messages from my body. There has certainly been a rise in Shakti energy for me whilst doing any form of womb work, I mentioned how fertility massage has this effect on me.

For those of you like me without wombs, Uma highlights how wonderful Womb Yoga can be as a healing and nurturing experience in the months and years following.

She also rightly states that, "the nurturing and creative energies of the womb space can resonate powerfully in the lives of women who no longer have wombs. The focus of yoga is on nurturing all dimensions of being, the vital energies as much as the physical body, and so the practices are absolutely nourishing for women post-hysterectomy: The engecti presence of the "yonist-hana," or space of homecoming, remains fully present even in the absence of the womb and/or ovaries, and so the practices of Womb Yoga can nourish all women."

In my experience thus far, and with the deep womb work beforehand and ritual around my surgery, I feel my womb space thankfully is still a powerful force!

YONI CARE TECHNIQUES

YONI IS A Sanskrit word for the female genitals, thought of as the source of all life and sacred and divine. So how can you take care of your yoni/vagina (insert your preferred word), especially if you have painful periods?

To keep the vagina healthy:

Soaps and most other products affect the PH level of the vagina and can cause irritation and bacterial vaginosis.

Do not wipe back to front. You must wipe front to back to avoid spreading bacteria.

Be aware of tampons and sanitary towels that have been bleached, I touched on this before. Also, be wary of toxic shock syndrome. You can choose cotton tampons or cloth pads or consider a menstrual cup; there are lots of options out there now.

Try not to wear tight clothing, and cotton knickers are more breathable than synthetic.

If you must take antibiotics, use probiotics so that you do not cause too much imbalance of bacteria in the vagina; this may also cause bacterial vaginosis, very common in women.

Be wary of scratching or anything that can cause bacteria to enter.

Castor oil packs—There are contraindications to using castor oil packs and caution is needed. Seek medical guidance from a doctor or physician to check if they are ok for you to use. Do not use if pregnant.

They are said to help with many things, including cysts, endometriosis, and circulation to the area (which may also have a positive effect on the lymph system). They were, for me, a very positive addition to my personal menstrual care routine and for adhesions post-surgery. I used organic castor oil.

Clare Spink (founder of fertility massage) offers her instructions on how to do a castor oil pack, as follows:

"A castor oil pack is an external application of castor oil. A piece of wool flannel is saturated in castor oil and applied to the abdomen with a hot water bottle or heat pack.

Instructions for use:

To Make the Pack: Use an old flannel, big enough to cover your abdominal area. Put it in a pan or bowl and pour warm castor oil on it. Saturate the whole flannel and leave it until it is well saturated. When you use it, you want it saturated, but not dripping. After each use, you will probably need to add a little more castor oil. You can use the flannel many times. When you're not using it, you can store it in a plastic box in the refrigerator or cool place.

Using the Pack:

- Use the pack in the evening, as you are resting before bed or when you have quiet time.

- Spread out a large plastic bag on the bed with an old towel on top so that the castor oil won't leak onto the bed. Fold a towel (that you will use only for castor oil packs, because the oil is almost impossible to wash out completely).

- Warm the heat pack/hot water bottle.

- Lie down on your back on the towel. Place the pack on your abdomen with the heating pad on top and the towel on top of that. It should be very warm, but not so hot it burns you.

- Ideally, keep the pack on for 1 to 1 ½ hours. Although anything from 20 minutes onwards is beneficial.

- Have a paper towel handy to wipe the oil off yourself when you get up.

- If you are trying to conceive, you can perform 3 times a week for a minimum of 30 minutes. Only perform during the first half of the menstrual cycle (from menstruation to ovulation)."

I also used an infrared red heating mat on my lower back which I found relaxed me and helped me to sleep, easing any discomforts. They are also said to help with stimulating blood flow and circulation. Again, please do your research and discuss with a medical doctor regarding whether they are safe for you to use. There are cautions and contraindications to these as well, as far as I know.

REGULAR SELF-CARE PRACTICE

SELF-CARE PRACTICES ARE now a vital part of my life rather than a luxury. I find I am happier all around with the kids and with work if I have taken time for myself. We are able to give more freely and easily when our own tank is full. Try to make it a priority, and you will see that you and the people in your life will be much better off for it.

I am able to fit in a regular daily practice now of ten to twenty minutes meditation or journaling either early morning or in the evening. I find that even after having a hysterectomy I use my hormonal shifts as a mindfulness practice to watch the rise and fall of hormones affecting how I interact with and perceive the world. I am able to check in daily to see what is arising in me or what wants to fall away. I try not to judge how I feel and am accepting of any changing emotions.

In meditation, I do the same as I learned to do when I trained to become a hypnobirthing teacher which is to breathe out for slightly longer than I breathe in. I start with four long slow counts in and six counts out. I like to imagine that I have a white light above the crown of my head, while breathing in, I take the white light into my body and let it clear any areas of tension. Then I breathe out and release it. You can say under your breath, "letting go" or "releasing tension" as you breathe out. You can do this anywhere, out shopping or standing in line at the su- permarket. If you feel stressed about the future or the past, then mindfulness is a great way to bring yourself back to the present. I also complete a body scan, checking all sensations from head to feet to bring myself back into the body. Since beginning men- strual cycle awareness, I find I have a closer connection to nature and the seasonal cycles as well.

I also realised that I was addicted to my phone and social media, as many of us are. I try to limit this now as much as pos- sible as well as watching the news. It's important to know what is going on in the world. But I found too much could leave you anxious with a very negative view of the world; perspective is important. Too much bombardment of fear-based news is not healthy. Balance it out; there are some amazing people doing amazing things in the world.

I am also a member of "*Rise Sister Rise*", a group created by the lovely Rebecca Campbell who is also author of the book of the same name. She has drawn in a group of amazing wom- en who are mostly working in spirituality, healing and creative industries and who are part of the rising feminine all over the world. This has been a fantastic group to be a part of. Rebecca updates monthly meditations or activation journeys and ritual ideas which has been a perfect adjunct to my healing and my own work with women.

A LOVE FOR THE FEMININE HEALING PLANT, CACAO

"CHOCOLATE IS A divine celestial drink, the sweat of the stars, the vital seed, divine nectar, the drink of the gods, panacea and universal medicine."

-Geronimo Piperni, quoted by Antonio Lavedán,
Spanish Army Surgeon, 1796

A true love of mine has been consuming ceremonial grade cacao after another series of synchronicities led me to a cacao ceremony. I had always been a huge fan of dark chocolate, but well-sourced ceremonial grade is not the same as the chocolate you buy from the shop. It is processed differently without the added sugar and fats. Much is sourced from South America, especially Peru and Guatemala where it is grown, harvested and fermented in a way that is said to maintain beneficial health properties.

I had seen an advertisement for a ceremony in London with Rebekah Shaman, author of *The Shaman's Last Apprentice*. I could not make any of the dates, so I just thought I would leave it for a while and then re-check at a later date to see if she had any new dates coming up.

A couple of months later whilst having a coffee in one of my local cafés, I could see a picture on the noticeboard of Rebekah. I literally had to do a double take. She was coming to my town to do a ceremony! I was getting used to "coincidences," but this felt very significant, and I booked straight on. It was a beautiful heart opening ceremony and from then on, I have taken a little bit of ceremonial grade cacao every day.

Most have heard of Ayahuasca as a powerful plant medicine, and ceremonial grade cacao is becoming very popular as a plant medicine and nutritional powerhouse in the UK. It is being used as an adjunct to any inner work or with meditation. The Aztecs and Mayans often used it in ceremony and ritual. Rebekah and others who do ceremony with cacao are always quick to point out it is not a psychedelic or anything like the effect of Ayahuasca.

It has been regarded as a feminine healing support, suppliers such as "Inner Guidance" who are a retreat centre in the UK include on their website (www.innerguidance.co.uk) a video of a cacao shaman discussing his purpose to share his love of the plant and the health benefits. You can buy the Guatemalan Raw Ceremonial Grade Cacao on their shop page. Scroll down below the cacao picture to watch the video (up at the time of writing). He describes it as a connector to whatever you want to connect to. Anything from a work activity to dancing or any creative project.

But his main reason for using it now is for the nutritional benefits. High grade cacao is said to have health benefits for the heart, especially for its magnesium and theobromine content. Be aware that it contains caffeine and could have adverse effects, check with a nutritionist first to see if it could benefit you. It is also said to have many antioxidants and is high ranking on the ORAC scale which stands for Oxygen Radical Absorbance Capacity, lab tests that attempt to measure the antioxidant capacity of different foods.

The magnesium benefit from cacao could help with period pain for women as many women are deficient in the mineral. The uterus is a muscle and a symptom of deficiency of magnesium is muscle cramps, therefore uterine cramps might be worse at menstruation if you are deficient. It is best to keep up your intake of magnesium. He does stress, as Rebekah does, that it shouldn't be taken in conjunction with antidepressants. You should never stop taking any medicine without consulting your doctor, and also let them know if you are taking any herbal remedies alongside medication in case they interact. I do feel that cacao was a huge support to me in my return back to health. I used it for the nutritional benefits and alongside meditation and journeying, and because I love the taste!

In ceremony with Rebekah, she also used the *Osho Zen Tarot* cards. We all took a card at the beginning of the ceremony and at the end. A few days later, I brought the pack. The focus being more on mindfulness and a reflection of how you can help yourself in the present moment. There is no emphasis on fortune telling, outcomes are changeable, and they connect you intuitively to the present moment to see if you can identify their message or guidance for you through connecting to your intuition, whatever is currently happening in your life. (I mentioned previously picking the "harmony card" with the dolphins surrounding my hysterectomy.) For the ceremony, we were all able to share and ascertain meaning for the card we pulled at the beginning and the end of the ceremony. The universe, it seemed, was continuing to guide me towards healing. My overall intuitive message from the ceremony was to prioritise certain areas of my life. Which I went on to do with great benefit.

Another beautiful way you can celebrate your menstrual cycle is with Moontime Chocolates, created by Milly in Devon in the UK. Milly attended the fertility massage course that I attended, and she has had her own journey towards the creation of her chocolates, which you can read about on her website (www. moontimechocolate.co.uk). Her chocolates are lovingly prepared for each stage of a woman's menstrual cycle, using herbs and ingredients that can support women in each phase. They are great to have in any ceremony or ritual, too. An example of one of her chocolates is Rose and Cramp Bark, which is my personal favourite! She describes them as…

"A soft and creamy truffle with rose to delight the feminine floral senses. A comforting taste to connect to your heart and womb. With a mild dose of cramp bark, to remind your muscles to relax and let the flow, flow."

Cramp bark is a traditional herbal remedy to ease menstrual cramps. It is "day 1" of her chocolate selection; she categorises them into cycle days, although of course if you have favourites you can eat them throughout the entire cycle. It's self-care after all! I love that she has looked at the ingredients and thoughtfully placed them for their benefits towards each phase.

NUTRITION, HERBS AND ESSENTIAL OILS.

WHILST DOING ALL the practices outlined in this book, I also investigated herbs, nutrition and essential oils, which all played their part in reducing symptoms. Due to my emergency operation and an infection, I had ended up taking around a month's worth of antibiotics as previously mentioned. This meant that as well as the bad bacteria, I would also be killing off the good in my digestive system. I feel this contributed to my poor health and exacerbation of endo at this time, especially as there has been a lot of research recently around the importance of a healthy gut. If you consider that a large proportion (over half) of your immune system is in your gut, imbalance of bad bacteria with not enough good can affect your health. With endo, it is important to have a healthy immune system. Probiotics, I would argue, are essential after a course of antibiotics. Your digestive system needs to be working well for it to absorb a wide range of nutrients. You may want to see a nutritionist to check if you need digestive enzymes, it would be frustrating if you are eating well but not able to absorb the nutrients you need.

Probiotics are not all created equal, and it is important that you take one that is proven to reach the areas of the gut the bacteria need to reach; they must be able to survive stomach acid. The BBC programme, "Trust Me, I'm a Doctor" set up an experiment in one of their episodes to research three different approaches towards increasing "friendly" bacteria in the gut. The results showed that consuming traditionally prepared and homemade goats milk kefir was the most effective at increasing bacteria strains in the gut (particularly lactobacillus) than the other options tested. Lactobacillus is thought to be good for general gut health. Chuckling Goat are an example of a company that uses the traditional methods. They also have a fantastic story and passion behind their brand, and I noticed a difference in my digestive health when I began using their products. They have a book, *The Kefir Solution: Natural Healing for IBS, Depression and Anxiety*. Keep in mind that most of your serotonin is made in the gut too, and so this might be affected with a damaged microbiome. This is why I also used it to overcome the health anxiety post birth after I had taken a month's worth of antibiotics. I believe this would have added to the problem as my gut was not in great health after that. If you suffer from endo, a recent article in *Psychologies Magazine* by Henrietta Norton, a registered nutritional therapist (wildnutrition.com), highlighted that beneficial bacteria can reduce an enzyme called beta-glucuronidase that remakes oestrogen in the gut and can contribute to oestrogen dominance, which is already dominant in most women with endo. Henrietta herself is passionate about nutritionally helping endo sufferers, as she was one herself.

Some women prefer to do a juice detox including herbal teas to give the digestive system a break if it is struggling but make sure you see a qualified nutritionist to do so safely or to see if it could personally help you. That goes for this entire chapter. This is what personally worked for me, but we are all unique. However, there are certain foods, herbs and supplements that can help us all with regard to endometriosis.

I also decided to try going vegan when reducing my endo symptoms. I wanted to avoid any processed food or any foods that could make the inflammation worse. My aim was to rebalance my hormones and help aid my body in its detoxification process, so foods or supplements to help this were key. I went organic to avoid adding the possibility of ingesting pesticides or chemicals.

Plants are packed with nutrients, so I was trying to help my body recover by not filling it with any junk or alcohol that would cause a flare or worsen symptoms. The jury is out on the use of antibiotics or hormones used in our animal products and how it affects our health after consumption. You can be an unhealthy vegan, so the key for me was to be predominantly plant based with all my food. Lots of vegetables and fruits, as well as nuts, seeds and legumes to ensure protein consumption. If this way of eating interests you, there are many vegan cookbooks, and restaurants are accommodating to the growing vegan population. I am currently in the process of developing an ebook of some of my favourite recipes that were beneficial for my endo.

Just pay attention to how foods make you feel if you have menstrual or health problems, and if you find certain foods trigger you, try avoiding them to see what results you get.

I was surprised how much I enjoyed the creativity involved in becoming vegan. It's amazing the range of plant-based foods out there and the combinations that taste fantastic. I found I was more creative in preparing food.

I also love essential oils; they are a part of my self-care kit. Geranium is said to be good for hormonal balance, but I never liked the smell. This is important when using oils. In some ways it is subjective, so if you decide you want to feel calm, sniff some oils and see which one you feel produces that effect in you.

For example, for many, lavender is relaxing and calming, but I find frankincense does this for me. Having said this, it is worth researching oils as they do have specific effects on the body relayed in scientific research. An aromatherapist will know the correct dilutions to massage into the body. It is important you follow the guidelines as too much will have a negative effect. You must also be aware of phototoxic oils that can increase your risk of sunburn. I find black pepper essential oil is great for aches and pains. Rose has a very feminine feel to me and is one of my favourite oils. I use it in an essential oil diffuser whilst having a bath. You can set a relaxing space with some music, dim the lights if possible and set the intention for connecting to the feminine receiving part of you.

You can also buy base creams which you can add to essential oils, and they are great to produce your own blend, but check whether your dilutions are safe.

On my mission to regain health, I also got rid of anything unnatural toiletry wise. If I couldn't eat it, I wouldn't put it on my body. Organic cold-pressed coconut oil has been my go-to skin cream.

I included as much Omega 3 fatty acids (anti-inflammatory) as I could from my diet with foods such as avocado. If you are not vegan, then oily fish is a fantastic source. I added the spice turmeric to much of my food due to its active compound curcumin, which is also regarded as anti-inflammatory. Endometriosis is an inflammatory condition.

I consumed lots of garlic. It stinks, but I haven't had a cold for ages! It is known to have a positive effect on the immune system. Ginger and peppermint capsules were my go-to for help in aiding digestion.

On my path to wellness, I regularly experimented with making smoothies to increase my nutritional intake. An example of two that I make and love are:

1 teaspoon Maca
1 teaspoon Spirulina
2 medjool dates
1 tablespoon raw cacao
1 banana
1 tablespoon tahini
1 cup of unsweetened almond milk
Blend.

A great protein smoothie that I love includes:
1 tablespoon almond butter
1 teaspoon chia seeds
1 cup hazelnut or unsweetened almond milk
1 teaspoon cacao
3 medjool dates
Strawberries or mango
Blend.

Some important vitamins and minerals that I increased after giving birth and having surgery included:

IRON - For menstruating women, it is important to make sure you are receiving enough iron. If on a vegan diet, then kale, spinach, beans and lentils can be useful sources but are better absorbed when taken with vitamin C, so you can have a kiwi fruit or some strawberries too. I was heavily anaemic after my haemorrhage and emergency operation and this truly affected my body. I took Spatone, which is a natural liquid iron supplement, as I found it easier on my digestive system than iron pills, but always check with your doctor first to see if you need to supplement as you may not need to.

VITAMIN D - This was important to me as there is a debate that deficiency is more common in people with chronic pain conditions. I know many people with certain diseases and discomforts feel better in summer or when the sun is shining. This was the case for me. I supplemented in winter, any deficiency in the body causes an imbalance, and with endometriosis, I wanted to give my body the best possible chance to heal. Vitamin D can have a positive effect on the immune system.

VITAMIN B12 - This is important as deficiency is said to cause tingling and pins and needles-type sensations and I certainly experienced this after the birth of my second child. It is worth having your levels checked if experiencing symptoms. I supplemented with B12 when going vegan.

I also used:

Peppermint oil - Indicated for IBS and bought in capsules. I used it for respiratory problems when I had pneumonia or any thoracic symptoms from endo; a couple of drops of the essential oil underneath my pillow at night helped me.

Ginger - Can be effective for nausea.

Cutting out dairy, refined sugar and gluten had a positive effect on my energy levels and hormonal balance. Sugar can wreak havoc on energy levels; spiking then lowering to where you crave more. Excess quantities of added sugar have been linked to inflammation and hormonal imbalance. Remember to check foods. Many processed foods and drinks can have high quantities. Regarding gluten, most people will be fine eating it, but it is interesting to note that there are many endo sufferers who find it beneficial on symptoms to cut it out. Some people are thought to have non-celiac gluten sensitivity. You can be tested if you feel it affects you after consumption.

I also became very aware of all the toxic household products I was using and anything I was putting on my body that could include dioxins that are linked to endo. I became aware of drinking pure or filtered water rather than tap to avoid any chemicals left in the water.

This is just a snapshot of what I did. As my symptoms improved, I added grass-fed organic meat and bone broth.

WARNING—DO NOT BECOME OBSESSIVE OVER FOOD!

DESPITE INCLUDING EVERYTHING I did to reduce my symptoms, please be aware of the implications of food obsession, and that includes "clean eating" (orthorexia), as it is known. We are all unique, and what affects my health may not be the same for you. If you do not have any menstrual conditions, then although it is always important to eat healthily, be aware of where you might be punishing yourself unnecessarily by not allowing certain foods which you might be ok with.

This is the same for someone with endo but most of us endo sufferers tend to be affected by what we eat, and it is beneficial for us to eat consciously for endo. There are so many of us that have reduced symptoms with proper nutrition. It's amazing how many treats you can eat that can be made healthy for endo, and it doesn't have to be a chore I have already said I loved the creativity involved and have created some amazing recipes that I may never have considered without changing my diet.

Unfortunately we are bombarded with social media and magazines showing images of airbrushed bodies, implying that we should all strive towards certain physical attributes. Never compare your body to anyone else's, it does an incredible job every day. It is unique to you; look after it, don't talk yourself down whilst looking in the mirror. Think about how miraculous your body is and what it does for you every day. It is not until something happens with regard to your health that you realise it really is the most important thing in our lives.

We again must question what we are being presented with and why. I also do not envy anyone in the media who feels they must put so much effort into looking a certain way or are made to put on a tonne of makeup before being placed in front of the camera. This is not great for self-esteem, for them or others. If you want to wear makeup because you love it and enjoy it, then great, go ahead, be creative. If it is because you somehow feel less without it, reflect on that and ask yourself, am I worried about what others will think? Do you use it as a mask to hide from the world? Take your power back; if that means expressing yourself with bright red lipstick, fire away.

I am sad about that year in my twenties when I reflect back, thinking about the risk of osteoporosis and the disrespect for the power and beauty of a body that has given me two beautiful boys. We must present a more truthful picture and love our bodies in all their shapes and sizes. They are incredible sources of wisdom and are miraculous in themselves. I am sure if I had connected to my body when younger, celebrated its cycles, and had positive body image education, I would have had the gratitude then that I have for my body today. We need to praise positive aspects of each other that are not based on physical looks. Particularly to help the younger generation, who are constantly receiving messages of body "perfection" as the aspiration to work towards. Remember our consumerist culture; there are many advertisements that want you to feel you will only be happy if you buy their products.

The irony is that the stress caused by all this pressure is more likely to cause issues and disconnect you from your true needs. Please don't self-sabotage; you are precious. Set boundaries on what messages you receive and take your power back. The aim is to feel healthy and happy in body, mind and spirit.

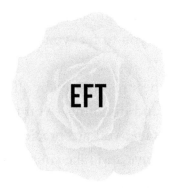

EFT

EFT (EMOTIONAL FREEDOM techniques) is often referred to as "psychological acupressure," or acupuncture without needles, and a focus on emotions. It is said to release blockages in the energy system which are the source of emotional pain or discomfort. It involves the use of your fingertips rather than needles to tap the end points of energy meridians under the skin.

Part of my journey to healing involved releasing old emotional wounds that I had not processed, particularly with beliefs formed in childhood. It amazed me in my sessions how an issue would arise that I had long forgotten about but had somehow played into a belief that I was still holding on to.

As children, we do not have the capacity to process emotions and so we can quickly form a belief from a negative experience.

For example:

"I cannot be loved unless (enter your story here!)"

"I have to do x, y, z in order to..."

"If I am nice, people will..."

And then enter the childhood experience that formed that belief.

For me, whilst healing past wounds, I actually felt like a small child again in the exact moment where I hadn't been able to release or process the pain. I was amazed at how powerful my emotions were, as if something had just happened that would cause the emotional charge. It truly felt like my inner child was releasing. I was able to comfort myself from an adult perspective and gain wisdom from the experience. I would usually feel much lighter after a session, too.

The areas that we tapped on included the inside of my right eyebrow, followed by the outside of the eyebrow, then onto the top of the lip, followed by the middle bottom section of the chin, the inner side of the collarbone, side of the ribs; karate chop outer side of the left hand.

You can do this on yourself repeating different statements relevant to the emotion you are wanting to release. For example, for use after surgery, you could repeat:

"Even though I feel anxious about my recovery, my body is healing beautifully inside."

You would tap on the points reading this sentence in full and then move on to the next one. You keep repeating the rounds and check what the emotional charge is on a scale of 1-10. You would ask this at the start of the tapping round and then at the end, note the difference in feeling. I was astounded by how effective it could be.

After the process, I would often journal. This is a great practice when doing any healing work. Not the same as a diary practice on what you did that day! I would often just write and see what came up for me. As part of the healing process, you can also do a letting-go ritual where you burn what you have written as part of the release of old unwanted emotions or energy.

A gratitude practice has also been high on my list of priorities. I spend a few minutes writing down a few things I am grateful for and it really helps to regain perspective if you are having a low day. You could also take gratitude pictures of moments in the year that you have been grateful for and, at the end of the year, create a gratitude photo book.

SOUND HEALING

I LOVE SOUND healing, and it is becoming very popular with sound baths cropping up all over the place at the moment. The use of gongs and crystal and Tibetan singing bowls produce some mesmerising sounds. It is also a great way to shift from your head into your body.

I find it shifts emotions and energy levels. If you are feeling tired, you may leave feeling energised or if you are feeling frustrated for some reason, you may find after that you are completely at peace; it's great if feeling overworked and stressed out.

Most people will have a very personal reaction with a sound bath, even though you can have many attending a session. The gongs can take you into deep relaxation. Some sound therapists contend that the vibrations of sound effect brainwaves producing a meditative and altered state. Those who lead workshops will not always know themselves what course the sound bath will take. It is often not rehearsed, as they feel into it intuitively.

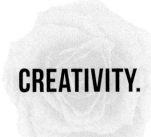

CREATIVITY.

I HAVE MENTIONED previously how my creativity has begun to flow in abundance. Creativity in any of the arts is renowned for its therapeutic benefits. I feel that moving out of my logical and rational mind into the creative and intuitive space has brought much happiness and been integral to healing. There is no surprise that we often call it the "healing arts." I began thinking about how I used to love painting when I was young, as most of us do when we are children. I had painted a picture in primary school that had been part of a school art competition at the village fete. It turned out that there was an artist there who owned a gallery and he ended up buying the painting I had created and hung it up in his gallery. I still have the photo of it in his gallery that he gave to my parents as he told them I should "keep painting." I did for a while because I loved it, but eventually I gave up as my practical logical side told me that it wouldn't lead me anywhere. I hadn't thought to keep going because I enjoyed it. Our conditioning can tell us that there are more important things than doing something purely for the love of it. There were times throughout my life when I felt the urge to paint again and I would for a while, but then I allowed other aspects of my life to take over.

I was also incredibly lucky that most of my twenties were spent doing creative projects involving theatre, dance or singing. Being on stage is also when I hit that sense of flow. I feel that when we are in this sense of flow we are tapping into our soul gifts.

Where are you currently creative in your life? Did you love being creative in the past?

If you feel you do not have time to be creative as you are too busy at work, or are a mum like me, or a single parent without much help, think about how you can reframe your experience to connect to creativity. You could do this through cooking a meal or painting with your kids; it does not have to be a separate practice. If you have children, then creating with them can be so much fun. They do not hold back from their creative essence. Our whole lives we are creating, whether in our jobs or in gardening or, in a larger sense, the way we live our lives.

If you are completely limited with time, then set the intention to notice how you can add creative touches to your day. How could you include more creativity in your work, for example? What could you do to make cooking dinner feel like an enjoyable creative process rather than a chore?

Is there anything that you could swap in your day to pursue a creative project instead? If you are a mum and usually watch television when the kids are asleep, could you do some painting or write your book? Which areas of creativity make you feel alive and in flow with the universe?

You may not see yourself as creative but we are all creative, we create our lives by our thoughts and the choices we make.

The joy of creativity is in that sense of play which we often lose as adults when responsibilities weigh heavily on our shoulders. We can still find many ways to keep that playful essence alive when we set the intention to connect to it. Many creatives feel connected to their soul or higher purpose when they are creating in flow with what lights them up. Think about what you loved doing as a child and start playing with it again. Your inner child will reward you for it with happiness.

RETURNING TO AUTHENTICITY

"CAN YOU REMEMBER who you were, before the world told you who you should be?"

-Danielle La Porte

I came across this quote from Danielle La Porte in her book, *The Fire Starter Sessions*. It resonated because I felt I had hidden parts of my authentic truth and inner desires for fear of judgement or ridicule. Through cyclic awareness and the healing modalities I was using I was being reconnected with the wisdom of the female body and mine had a lot to say—I could no longer hide.

You may have different parts of yourself that you have denied and there will be relevance and power in you reclaiming them.

I always loved travelling. It was regularly exciting, and I spent a lot of time living and working abroad and meeting fascinating people. I was always curious and found myself doing many things related to performing and I even became a muse to artists in Australia at one point! I was also part of an astrology group for a while as I was interested in the healing arts and spirituality. I didn't have many endo or period problems at this time of my life, which could be due to the fact that I was living in my authenticity and was connecting to my soul passions and I rarely felt stressed.

The problem came when I returned "home" to the UK and I did what so many of us do. I got lost in the world of "shoulds" and became a school teacher because I felt that was acceptable, in the sense that it is a "sensible job." Others had often asked when I would settle down and get a "real job" and I stopped listening to my own feelings around how I wanted to live my life.

It is so important that we tap into our own heart and truth. We do not have to follow paths we feel are acceptable in the eyes of others if they are not what we truly desire. The world needs you to be unique and offer your unique gifts.

I'd also wanted to emigrate to Australia, and teaching could have given me the qualifications and points to go. Not a great reason to expend that much effort on training! There were many aspects of training and teaching that I did love and I'm grateful for the many skills I've obtained, but I remember standing in my classroom one day thinking, how did I end up here?

It was never my dream after years of living abroad and the plans I had for myself to end up back in school. I was not living in the truth of what I wanted for myself. I had always had jobs that involved travel and excitement and a sense of freedom. The way I liked to live was unique to me. Many others like to work in this way too, and many don't. Again, the point is, are you living in truth with your soul and passions? Does your work motivate you or does it drain you?

I had harboured a dream to work for myself and so this is finally what I did. I decided to pursue holistic therapies. I now realise it was a pertinent move considering what later ensued.

My spiritual curiosity seemed to ignite again after ten years of not connecting to this part of myself, the catalyst being the trauma after birthing my second child. I certainly wasn't expecting to reunite this curiosity from the experience.

What I now know to be quite common is that the experience after giving birth had caused me to have a surge of creative energy. I found myself planning what the next steps would be with my work. The sacral chakra (below navel/reproductive space for women) is said to be active still after birth. Having done all my womb work, I now clearly see correlations in my own life in how this space affects my creativity. This only happened in those first few months before the pain started.

I kept mulling over ideas, and reiki was one of them to further my therapy offerings to clients. I remember writing different options on pieces of paper, screwing them up and choosing one, like flipping a coin, because there were so many options I wanted to take. I tried a best out of three and chose reiki every time. So, I searched online for a reiki master near me. If I'm honest, I didn't think it would have that much of an effect on me. I wasn't even sure if I believed in it, but I found a beautiful reiki master, Melanie Pitman. I booked her private training day. When I met her, she was so bubbly, and we hit it off straight away. It felt like we had already known each other for years.

In the first initiation, I do not remember feeling much afterwards, but the second, I did. This was the very first time I encountered the visual of the Native American. I could see clearly in my mind his headdress, full of feathers, and he had an eagle with him. I felt he represented a shaman.

Afterwards when we went upstairs, I remember Melanie asking me if I was ok. I think I was a little shell shocked; something had shifted energetically, I felt it in my body. Mel, of course, was used to this as she does a lot of energy work. What ensued in the following few weeks was not easy as I was feeling very sensitive to the energy of others around me. Those of you who are empaths will know it can be difficult sometimes as well as a gift.

Looking back, I see that it was interesting that I found her when I did. It was the start of many synchronistic encounters. Lots of people say that reiki finds you when you need it. In hindsight, there were many choices that I was making to help others that inadvertently ended up helping me. I was being shown the importance of putting myself first so that I could be truly present for others. I was ignoring my needs by trying to avoid looking at my own pain around the trauma I didn't want to acknowledge.

I remember when doing reiki on myself that I kept being drawn to my womb area. It wasn't until a few months later when my 'periods' returned after breastfeeding that I had realised there were real problems after the retained placenta and following operation. I highlighted previously that endometriosis symptoms can disappear whilst pregnant or breastfeeding and this is what happened with me.

When I was a child I was often told that I had a very "vivid imagination." I lost this as I grew up as many of us do when the rational and logical mind are praised and valued. I think a strong imagination is a blessing, especially for creative and artistic pursuits. But it's also important to feel with your heart and body in order to access information about what wants to be acknowledged within you.

I always found I could read people quickly, sensing what others were feeling or thinking without them saying a word; a sort of sixth sense. It was only when I had this pointed out to me that not everyone has this ability, that I realised it may be a gift as well as difficult to deal with sometimes. I later knew that I could take on other people's energy, feeling how they felt, and realised it is part of being an empath. Which is a good thing in the work I do but can make you sensitive to negativity where it's easy to feel others' emotions as if they are your own. If for example someone has just had an argument I can sense it clearly. We all have these abilities but it seems some of us are more sensitive or reactive to it.

This is where I had to learn to put boundaries in place to protect myself. This did not mean that I became uncaring. I was able to give out energetically when I wasn't drained myself.

Where do you need to place boundaries in your life? If you are an empath, it is important to not take the pain of others as your own. We can hold space and support with more ease when we are at ease and grounded in ourselves. I found this very important on my path back to wellness. I suffered if I did too much, or if I felt obliged to do something to keep others happy. It became really important. We must utilise our energy and listen to our bodies; that means learning to say no when you need time out. Sometimes, as empaths, we can lose sense of what is and isn't ours. We can expend a lot of energy trying to make others happy, as their energy can impact us if we are not rooted in ourselves. If we acknowledge that, we can remain centred despite what others are feeling.

Being aware and expressing our authentic truths in the moment and setting boundaries is paramount to our wellbeing. It's far more exciting and interesting when we encourage our uniqueness rather than try to hide it in order to fit in. Fearing others' judgements and hiding your truth means likeminded souls can't find you; you give your power away by worrying too much about the opinions of others. You live with you. Time is short; do what makes you happy. If friends and family don't like it or criticize you, don't take it to heart and accept that not everyone will agree with you. Move forth in your truth anyway.

WISDOM OBTAINED

I FOUND THAT self-love and care were instrumental in re-
gaining my health after the postnatal surgery and proceeding
endo issues. I always thought I would need to "fight" to regain
my health, and there is a time when we may have to fight to
receive appropriate care, but love and acceptance played a huge
role. Choosing love over fear and having that awareness provided nuggets of wisdom. When my challenging year happened, I
played the "why me?" card but also actually may have received
some answers to that question, and, of course, sometimes sh**
happens. It is how we deal with what happens to us that makes
the difference. It may sound like an old cliché, but many truths
are. I worked with myself and my cycle and reduced symptoms.
If you love and look after yourself, you can relate to other aspects of your life with love and more ease. The support I received
from being in circle, doing rituals, womb massage, rebozo, and
journeying with Menstrual Medicine Circle's accelerated my
understanding of the wisdom of the female body and was instrumental in my healing process. Any negative or false beliefs I
held were made conscious through doing this inner work. Particularly regarding the collective and individual shame we hold

as women. I could really sense my bodies messages the more I tuned in to them.

Let's celebrate women and our transitions through the life phases; the landscape is less scary when the territory is explored and shared. Question where any shame comes from, change can't happen unless we begin to speak out. It's great to see women raising awareness of subjugation. The recent #MeToo campaign that went viral online is a great example. With Reese Witherspoon in her speech at the Golden Globes stating that she hates receiving scripts with a woman turning to a man when in trouble, asking, "What are we going to do?" as if women wouldn't know and need to ask men to decide. Language carries meaning—it's time to call it out.

I wouldn't have the wisdom and courage to stand by my authenticity if it wasn't for exploring my shadows and unhealed wounds. It is sometimes through our pain that we discover our power. It is through our vulnerability that we can find our truth and connection to our heart, and in return, true connection to others. Without hiding behind our masks or roles in life.

In order to heal, we must feel it all. I realised that through trauma we switch a part of us off, closing off our emotions and disengaging from our bodies in order to not feel pain or rejection. A natural response mostly. The trouble is, if we close off the pain, we risk closing off all of our other emotions too. In my experience and with that of my clients we become numb in trying to protect ourselves, feeling lost with no map or directions on how to get back. This is often when life, (insert preferred word) may step in. For me, I felt I was guided to work with my womb and cyclic wisdom as this was where I needed to find healing.

But I had to surrender first, letting go of the reigns and allowing the space for life to guide me.

We must find the courage and support to feel it all at some point, otherwise we are not truly alive and living to our potential. If we want to feel the highs, we must feel the lows. It really is ok not to feel ok. We make judgements of what is positive or negative based on our past experiences. What is viewed as negative for one person might be positive for another.

We have a range of emotions for a reason. And there can be gifts and wisdom in the lows if we look for the meaning or messages.

It is not uncommon for any of us to experience a trauma, illness or grief that propels us into an emotional storm and makes us question everything in our lives. I now see that this destruction can turn out to be a blessing or a soul calling, a chance to really prioritise and to be honest with ourselves about who we truly are and what we really want; a chance to start over and empower yourself, an opportunity to transmute fear into love, to reconnect with a deeper respect for yourself. You do not need to have had a trauma or any significant incident happen for you to reawaken to this.

My unexpected quest had also led me to question many of my beliefs and helped me to see where I had given my power away and disowned some of my passions and desires for fear of judgement and ridicule.

Allow space so that creativity and life can move you, opening up to that sense of flow. Where we are observing the events and remain in awe of the outcomes, like artists who produce work and step back mesmerised by the creations that have expressed themselves through them. When we are in a state of trying to control life, this flow gets blocked, it has no access and we struggle, wanting things to go our way. What if the life we plan and strive so hard for is not as good as what life has in store for us, if we allowed it to unfold? Are you not allowing the room and space for opportunities to emerge or inspiration to come?

What if we are fighting against life, trying to please others or fit ourselves into a box that our families or friends accept, or that fits their wants and wishes for us but not ours? What if what we believe is true about this, is not actually true?

Are you in a relationship you love? Are you doing a job that makes you want to get up in the morning? Are you passionate? Are you connected to your body and sensuality? Are you free? Are you judging yourself and others?

As women, we can feel guilty about self-love and care because of a conditioning or judgement that it is selfish; trust me, it's not. You want to thrive, not survive. You can give far more freely and easily when your tank is full. The feminine is about receiving, how does this make you feel? Boundaries are necessary to protect your energy and emotional state; it's ok to say no.

Are you a perfectionist? I suffered with this one in the past. It is not a good trait. I have also been completely carefree and found it much more fulfilling. If you have this tendency, you will never be satisfied or feel that anything is good enough; it's good to learn to let go. We do not need perfection in order to thrive. It may be a great trait for an employer or from a work perspective, but it is the constant striving that can cause emotional and mental unrest and disharmony. Where in your life do you have this trait?

Perfectionism is often tied up with self-worth, you do not need to prove yourself to anybody. I have discovered with clients that it can often be there because a parent or family member constantly criticized and made their child feel as if they were never good enough. Whether this was intentional or not, it is always unobtainable, and the goal posts will always move. Happiness comes from accepting all of yourself, including any perceived "imperfections."

Our bodies are incredible at healing and keeping us going without us having to think or control anything, but if we keep piling up the cr**, whether emotional, physical or mental, we could start drowning in it all and it could manifest physically as dis-ease. We must respect the beauty of our body that holds so much wisdom; self-love and care can hold the power to change the course of how we experience ourselves and our lives.

On the other side of the coin, when illness or trauma happen, or events are out of your control, you can find your way home to yourself. There is light when you look for it. Of course, feel the anger or sadness and move through the pain. But ultimately, love, self-care, surrendering and outside support can offer a return to wellness.

Write in your journal. What do you feel passionate about and love? Do you have enough of this in your life? How can you get more of it?

The trauma I experienced caused me to reflect on my life. I knew that there was transformation on its way from a healing perspective. I have said the quest was unexpected and that is maybe why I fell in love with it all the more, eventually, when I had learned its lessons and trusted that I was where I needed to be.

I've never been one to plan, and I've always loved spontaneity and adventure, and although it was the most difficult time of my life, I reconnected with myself; life began to flow again as I let go of a need to control as so many of us do. A deeper part of me wanted to be heard. I was being asked to grow and transform from it all and was being reminded of the pieces of the puzzle of my own life fitting together to show me the next steps I could take.

For happiness, do not compare your situation to anyone else's. We all go through the highs and lows of life at some stage and your journey is truly your own, just as your lessons and your passions are your own, too. Stick to your truths. It is far easier to flow with life than fight against it.

You can begin your self-care and menstrual (or lunar) cycle tracking journey in the last pages of this book.

Thank you for reading until the end. I would be so grateful for an Amazon review if it has helped you or sparked your curiosity. I would love your feedback. Please share with those you feel could benefit. Leaving a review really will help other women to find this book. You can also follow my journey on my blog and discover my online and workshop offerings on the magic and power of charting and flowing with your menstrual cycle (as well as tips for menstrual conditions and pain) at melanierossiter.com. I truly teach what I wish I'd known and what every woman should know. You will find Womb Yoga and most of the other modalities I discuss on my site and in my community of women.

Much love sister

BIBLIOGRAPHY

Campbell, Rebecca. (2016). *Rise Sister Rise: A Guide to Unleashing the Wise, Wild Woman Within*. London, UK: Hay House. rebeccacampbell.me

Diamont, Anita. (1997). *The Red Tent*. New York: St Martin's Press.

Dinsmore-Tuli, Uma (2013*) Yoni Shakti: A Woman's Guide to Power and Freedom Through Yoga and Tantra*. London, UK: Pinter and Martin.

Dinsmore-Tuli (2008) *Teach Yourself Yoga for Pregnancy and Birth*. London, UK: Hodder Education.
www.umadinsmoretuli.com
yonishakti.co
wombyoga.org
yoganidanetwork.org

Gray, Miranda. (2009). *Red Moon*. London, UK: Fastprint Gold. mirandagray.co.uk

Jones, Shann Nix. (2018). *The Kefir Solution: Natural Healing for IBS, Depression and Anxiety*. London, UK: Hay House.

Kent, Tami Lynn. (2011). *Wild Feminine: Finding Power, Spirit & Joy in the Female Body*. Atria Books/Beyond Words. wildfeminine.com

La Porte, Danielle. (2012). *The Fire Starter Sessions*. London, UK: Hay House. DanielleLaPorte.com

Lister, Lisa. (2017). *Witch, Unleashed. Untamed. Unapologetic*. London, UK: Hay House.

Lister, Lisa (2016) *Love Your Lady Landscape: Trust Your Gut, Care for 'Down There' and Reclaim Your Fierce and Feminine SHE Power* London, UK: Hay House lisalister.com

Norman, Abby. (2018). *Ask Me About My Uterus: A Quest to Make Doctors Believe in Women's Pain*. New York: Nation Books.

Pope, Alexandra and Wurlitzer, Sjanie Hugo. (2017). *Wild Power*. London, UK: Hay House. redschool.net

Shaman, Rebekah. (2013). *The Shaman's Last Apprentice: The Story of a Modern Day Urban Shaman*. London, UK: Amaru 2nd Edition rebekahshaman.com

Zen, Osho. Padma, Deva. (2016) *Osho Zen Tarot: The Transcendental Game of Zen: 79 Cards Plus Instruction Book*: New York: St Martin's Press.

Kindred Spirit Magazine- www.kindredspirit.co.uk
Psychologies Magazine- www.psychologies.co.uk

Thanks to…
Clare Spink- fertilitymassage.co.uk
Leora Leboff-auramama.co.uk
Andrea Clarke- mamaquillafertility.com

A SPECIAL THANK YOU

A SPECIAL THANK you to my husband Sam Rossiter and also to Leora Leboff, Tammy Driver and Clare Spink. But much love to all of you who were involved in my journey either directly or inadvertently.

MENSTRUAL CYCLE DAY
(DAY 1 = FIRST DAY OF YOUR PERIOD)
MOON PHASE

Energy Levels

Self-Care Intentions

Prominent Feelings/Emotions

What I Need to Release/Let Go Of

Where I Need to Set Boundaries

What I am Grateful For Today

MENSTRUAL CYCLE DAY
(DAY 1 = FIRST DAY OF YOUR PERIOD)
MOON PHASE

Energy Levels

Self-Care Intentions

Prominent Feelings/Emotions

What I Need to Release/Let Go Of

Where I Need to Set Boundaries

What I am Grateful For Today

MENSTRUAL CYCLE DAY
(DAY 1 = FIRST DAY OF YOUR PERIOD)
MOON PHASE

Energy Levels

Self-Care Intentions

Prominent Feelings/Emotions

What I Need to Release/Let Go Of

Where I Need to Set Boundaries

What I am Grateful For Today

MENSTRUAL CYCLE DAY
(DAY 1 = FIRST DAY OF YOUR PERIOD)
MOON PHASE

Energy Levels

Self-Care Intentions

Prominent Feelings/Emotions

What I Need to Release/Let Go Of

Where I Need to Set Boundaries

What I am Grateful For Today

MENSTRUAL CYCLE DAY
(DAY 1 = FIRST DAY OF YOUR PERIOD)
MOON PHASE

Energy Levels

Self-Care Intentions

Prominent Feelings/Emotions

What I Need to Release/Let Go Of

Where I Need to Set Boundaries

What I am Grateful For Today

MENSTRUAL CYCLE DAY
(DAY 1 = FIRST DAY OF YOUR PERIOD)
MOON PHASE

Energy Levels

Self-Care Intentions

Prominent Feelings/Emotions

What I Need to Release/Let Go Of

Where I Need to Set Boundaries

What I am Grateful For Today

MENSTRUAL CYCLE DAY
(DAY 1 = FIRST DAY OF YOUR PERIOD)

MOON PHASE

Energy Levels

Self-Care Intentions

Prominent Feelings/Emotions

What I Need to Release/Let Go Of

Where I Need to Set Boundaries

What I am Grateful For Today

MENSTRUAL CYCLE DAY
(DAY 1 = FIRST DAY OF YOUR PERIOD)
MOON PHASE

Energy Levels

Self-Care Intentions

Prominent Feelings/Emotions

What I Need to Release/Let Go Of

Where I Need to Set Boundaries

What I am Grateful For Today

Printed in Great Britain
by Amazon

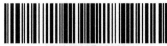

87190529R00099